Business Co

Healthcare Providers: A Quick Reference for Midwives, NPs, PAs, CNSs and other Disruptive Innovators

Joan Slager, CNM, MSN

Director, Nurse-Midwifery
Bronson Women's Service
Kalamazoo, Michigan

JONES AND BARTLETT PUBLISHERS

Sudbury, Massachusetts

BOSTON TORONTO LONDON SINGAPORE

World Headquarters
Jones and Bartlett Publishers
40 Tall Pine Drive
Sudbury, MA 01776
978-443-5000
info@jbpub.com
www.jbpub.com

Jones and Bartlett Publishers Canada
2406 Nikanna Road
Mississauga, ON L5C 2W6
CANADA

Jones and Bartlett Publishers International
Barb House, Barb Mews
London W6 7PA
UK

Library of Congress Cataloging-in-Publication Data

Slager, Joan.
Business concepts for healthcare providers: A quick reference for midwives, nps, pas, cnss and other disruptive innovators / Joan Slager.—1st ed.
p. ; cm.
Includes bibliographical references and index.
ISBN 0-7637-2290-1 (pbk.)
1. Managed care plans (Medical care)—Handbooks, manuals, etc. 2. Medicine—Practice—Finance—Handbooks, manuals, etc. 3. Medical economics—Handbooks, manuals, etc.
[DNLM: 1. Practice Management—organization & administration—Handbooks. 2. Managed Care Programs—Handbooks. 3. Organizational Innovation—Handbooks. W 49 S631c 2004] I. Title.
RA413.S535 2004
362.1'04258—dc22

2003022256

Acquisitions Editor: Penny M. Glynn
Production Manager: Amy Rose
Associate Production Editor: Jenny L. McIsaac
Editorial Assistant: Amy Sibley
Marketing Manager: Joy Stark-Vancs
Marketing Associate: Elizabeth Waterfall
Manufacturing Buyer: Amy Bacus
Cover Design: Bret Kerr
Composition: Interactive Composition Corporation
Printing and Binding: Malloy Inc.
Cover Printing: Malloy Inc.

Printed in the United States of America
07 06 05 04 03 10 9 8 7 6 5 4 3 2 1

Dedication

This book is dedicated to Eunice K. Ernst, CNM, MPH, FACNM, my first (and most demanding) business instructor and to Vern, Michele, Mark and Meredith for always being the wind beneath my wings.

TABLE OF CONTENTS

PREFACE

This book was written for the non-physician healthcare provider; that often misunderstood, mislabeled member of the healthcare team.

As a non-physician provider for the past 12 years, it has been my observation that my colleagues, while being well prepared to provide excellent clinical care, are ill-equipped in matters of business. Such ignorance has resulted in inadequate compensation, inappropriate restriction, and unfair representation of the non-physician provider. Ultimately, jobs are lost and practices have closed depriving the families we serve of the quality healthcare they deserve.

This book is intended to be a "pocket consult" for the non-physician provider who wishes to gain a basic understanding of some of the most common concepts of the business of being a healthcare provider. At the end of the book there are 'Suggested Readings' which will direct the reader to a more comprehensive study of the topic.

Much of the material in this book is derived from personal experience. As a service director for a large nurse-midwifery service, the "concepts of business" learned over the past few years have given me insights that I hope to pass on to you, the reader, with the hope that it may lead to the development of successful, thriving, savvy healthcare providers and practices.

So, you are now a nurse-practitioner, nurse-midwife, clinical nurse specialist, physician's assistant, nurse anesthetist, etc. You have been educated, observed, evaluated, examined, and certified. Congratulations! You now can begin paying back all of those student loans and begin doing what you have been educated to do. Or can you?

For some, employment (and patients) have been waiting for you to finish. For others the future is somewhat less certain. Either way, the average healthcare provider enters the work force well prepared for clinical challenges, but somewhat less schooled in the common aspects of business.

Education programs are already overloaded with the amount of clinical knowledge that must be part of a curriculum, leaving precious little time for teaching students basic business concepts. The student, in turn, is more interested in mastering clinical skills than researching state licensure rules and regulations.

Non-physician healthcare providers have been around awhile. Why the knowledge deficit? Historically, non-physician healthcare professionals have been employees of physician practices, hospital clinics, and community health centers. As an employee, the provider was paid a salary and benefits for working for the employer. In fact, many of these providers were originally employed by the practice and sent to school in order to take on additional responsibilities. For such "employees," business concepts were of little concern.

Other providers were educated and recruited to address a specific public health need. They too were concerned more with meeting the challenges of their patient populations with little concern for productivity and benchmarking.

As healthcare continues to evolve, and as healthcare professionals continue to meet today's clinical challenges, they are now faced with demonstrating knowledge of things such as fiscal responsibility, productivity, and quality management. Failure to develop business acumen may result in lost jobs, closing practices or becoming subjected to unreasonable demands or expectations.

Non-physician healthcare providers may also opt to become entrepreneurs. No longer content with simply being employed by a clinic or physician practice, or forced to create his or her own opportunity for practice, this provider is faced with the many challenges of self-employment as well as developing a practice. Whatever the background or motivation, this book is designed to be a primer in business for the non-traditional healthcare provider.[1]

[1]In this book, for purposes of clarification, the term *clinician* refers to non-physician providers generically. The term *healthcare provider* refers to both physician and non-physician providers.

INTRODUCTION

The healthcare crisis facing this country has reached epidemic proportions. The appearance of the non-physician provider in this country is due, in part, to the crisis. The non-physician provider (nurse practitioner, nurse-midwife, physician assistant, clinical nurse specialist, nurse anesthetist, etc.) is often utilized in underserved areas, providing care to indigent populations as a solution to the problem of access, to care. More recently, physician practices and healthcare organizations have employed these professionals in efforts to increase productivity and revenue.

While the quality of care provided by the non-physician provider has been well documented,[1] and patients are accepting these providers with a high degree of satisfaction, established, traditional medicine still maintains a tight hold on the control of the practice of the non-physician provider.

Christensen, Bohmer and Kenagy, in their article entitled, *Will Disruptive Innovations Cure Health Care?,*[2] suggest that the non-physician healthcare provider is part of the solution to the healthcare crises facing the country today. These highly trained, competent individuals are able to provide the majority of healthcare to the majority of people at reasonable cost. The high cost, high tech procedures, and professionals should be utilized to care for the small majority of individuals that require such expertise. Employing non-physician providers, as the primary providers of healthcare, is *innovative* but *disruptive* to the traditional healthcare delivery system. Thus the term: *disruptive innovators.*

While strategically well placed to accept the challenge of becoming *disruptive innovators,* the average non-physician provider is ill-prepared in the concepts of business that ultimately lead to the success of such a venture. It is with this in mind that this book was written.

[1]Expanding Roles of Nurse Practitioners and Physician's Assistants, Position Paper, American College of Physicians-American Society of Internal Medicine; January 22, 2000.

MacDorman MF, Singh GK. Midwifery care, social and medical risk factors, and birth outcomes in the USA. *J Epidemiol Community Health* 1998; 52:310–317.

[2]Christensen, Clayton M., Bohmer, Richard, and Kenagy, John, "Will Disruptive Innovations Cure Health Care?", *Harvard Business Review,* Sept.–Oct. 2000.

ACKNOWLEDGEMENTS

"Know what you are worth" insisted Kitty Ernst, CNM, MPH, FACNM to a group of fledgling nurse-midwifery students in the spring of 1991. Just as I will never forget my first night's sleep on a real feather bed on a farm in Pennsylvania, I could not forget those early lessons in business spoken by one of the most *disruptive innovators* I have ever had the privilege to know. The seeds were planted and many others have participated in the feeding and watering of them.

My "business" career began with lecturing on the topics of billing and coding at the Midwifery Business Institute in the fall of 1999. Lisa Kane-Low, CNM, PhD, FACNM, Carol Williams, MS, RNC, and Patricia Crane Cyr, CNM, MSN, with others, created a forum where nurse-midwives could learn aspects of business not taught in basic education programs. At the third annual Midwifery Business Institute, I had suggested a presentation on billing and coding as a future topic which resulted in me being scheduled to present a series of lectures on the subject the follow year.

While researching and preparing for those presentations, I developed a personal interest in applying what I had learned in order to improve the billing practices within my own service. The midwifery service in which I worked became the largest and one of the most financially successful practices in Michigan. Additionally, it became painfully clear that the majority of healthcare providers are ignorant of billing and other business concepts, sometimes jeopardizing their jobs or placing their practices at risk for closing. I wish to express my thanks to the Certified Nurse-Midwives of Bronson Women's Service who worked to build the strong practice that it is, and to all of the *disruptive innovators* who strive for competence in business in addition to clinical excellence.

It has also been my pleasure to work with and learn from excellent, collaborative physicians and innovative and supportive administrators. All *disruptive innovators* should be so fortunate. The road to success for the *disruptive innovator* at times seems to travel mostly up hill and it is to our good fortune when our physician colleagues and administrators help rather than hinder our efforts to become productive and autonomous members of the healthcare team.

The impetus for writing the book came from Kerri D. Schuiling, CNM, PhD, a colleague and dear friend who never runs out of energy. As Dean of the School of Nursing of Northern Michigan University, Kerri saw a need for a resource that new clinicians could use to assist with their introduction to the world of business. The pep talks and cheerleading always came at just the right time.

A special thanks to Jennifer Moore, RN, Eric Dyson, and Laura Benthin for providing valuable feedback, and a very special thanks to Marion McCartney, CNM, who not only provided feedback for this book, but has always given sound business advice and provided crisis intervention to clinicians in need.

I am most grateful to my good friend, Edward Annen, Jr., for agreeing to author the chapter on contracting and for providing substance and validity to the liability chapter.

There are others who have been responsible for my education in business, without whom I would have been unprepared to direct a large CNM practice or write a book on business. These women have been colleagues, mentors and friends and have taught me much: Cathy Collins-Fulea, MSN, CNM, FACNM, Helen Gordon, MS, CNM, Carolyn Gegor, MS, CNM, RDMS, FACNM, Barbara Hughes, MS, MBA, CNM, Jan Kriebs, CNM, MSN, FACNM, Nancy Jo Reedy, MS, CNM, MPH, and Deanne Williams, MS, CNM, FACNM.

On the home front, I give my undying love and gratitude to my friends who keep me on track providing wit and wisdom, to God who sustains me, and to my family whose unfailing love and support allows me to keep all of the plates spinning.

Joani Slager

CHAPTER 1

A CRISIS IS AN OPPORTUNITY

Once their education program has been completed, most healthcare providers are faced with converting what they have learned into earning a living. The traditional healthcare provider (a physician) felt called into service, completed an education program, and then hung up a shingle and began to practice. The physician enjoyed status in the community, a higher standard of living, and was held in reverence by his patients. No one questioned "the doctor." The doctor, in return, selflessly served his patients nearly 24 hours a day, 7 days a week.

The path is somewhat less clear for the nonphysician provider. He or she may anticipate being hired by an organization, a physician's office, or a community health center. The nonphysician provider may look forward to starting his or her own business. Whatever the case, the nonphysician provider should keep in mind that a crisis may be just the opportunity he or she is looking for to enter the workforce, open a practice, or increase his or her value to an organization. This chapter will discuss various crises that have historically presented opportunities to clinicians.

HISTORICAL BACKGROUND

One of the first "crises" to strike healthcare delivery was the lack of care for rural and inner-city populations; what we have come to call the "underserved." Although rural areas were sometimes served by a "country doctor," many people in remote areas were often without health care. Alternatives to traditional health care began to evolve to meet the needs of underserved communities. Public health nurses played a large role in caring for the country's inner-city and rural populations. During times of war, nurses and medics became the front-line healthcare providers.

Mary Breckenridge, a nurse, recruited the first nurse-midwives (educated in England) to address the issue of infant and maternal mortality, due to the unavailability of care providers for women, in the mountains of eastern Kentucky.[1] Similarly, after the Vietnam War Navy corpsmen who had received medical training during the war became the first physician's assistant students at Duke University Medical Center in North Carolina in the mid-1960s in response to a shortage of primary care physicians.[2]

Other, more recent, changes in health care have greatly altered traditional practice. Financial strains, managed care, medical liability, and the disappearance of fee-for-service billing have changed the way healthcare providers can and do practice. More women have entered medicine in the last two decades than all other decades combined,[3] and because these women also wanted families, the physician's job description and requirements for selflessness began to be questioned. Managed care has greatly influenced changes in the healthcare delivery system as providers were asked to do more with less, forcing them to discover more efficient ways to provide care.

Today, enrollment in medical schools is down; medical students are watching their contemporaries finish school and earn a living while they haven't even completed half of their education.[4] The physician is no longer viewed with the same reverence as in the past, liability insurance poses an immense expense, as well as a threat to practice; and the debt-to-income ratio of physicians continues to climb. These trends are creating crises, and therefore lots of opportunity for the **disruptive innovator**.

Many legislators and physicians oppose and create barriers to practice for nonphysician clinicians, fearing the development of a two-tiered health system (only the rich see physicians). Consider a two-tiered health system where the healthy and those with routine acute illnesses are treated by nonphysician providers, leaving the management of complex problems and the employment of costly technology to highly trained physicians.

In their article *Will Disruptive Innovations Cure Health Care?*, Christensen et al.[5] point out that the highly specialized technological advances in health care only benefit a small segment of the population; however, the cost of delivering these services is disproportionately large. They suggest that disruptive innovators who are trained to recognize and treat common problems are a much more cost-effective way to deliver health care to the majority of people. Christensen et al. also suggest that if the healthcare system was redesigned based on a model of care that used entry-level providers, the system would be more cost-effective and efficient. Improved access to care could also be anticipated.

In examining ways to solve the various healthcare crises, legislators are aggressively searching for ways to solve the problem of delivering quality health care to all persons. Among the recurrent themes defining the ideal healthcare delivery system are accessibility, quality, health promotion and wellness, and lower costs. Adopting a model of care that employs disruptive innovators as primary care providers would enable these themes to be incorporated. The healthcare crisis of today is an opportunity for tomorrow's career development.

CRISES

The following are a number of potential crises that can result in opportunities for the clinician today.

Crisis: Cost

Nonphysician providers are educated in one third to one half the time it takes to educate a physician and at roughly one fourth the cost. Nonphysician providers can generate revenue that greatly exceeds the cost of their salaries, benefits, and liability insurance.

The lower cost of education and the shorter time it takes to achieve certification and licensure makes the clinician an attractive option for employers. Some clinicians are fortunate enough to have been sponsored by future employers who paid for all or part of their educational expenses, expecting in return a commitment from the clinician for an agreed upon amount of service. Such arrangements may appear attractive at the onset, but the clinician would be wise to consider alternative funding and be aware of the risks and benefits of such an agreement.

Receiving financial assistance from a potential employer can alleviate some of the stress of leaving the workforce to return to school. In addition, the clinician is assured employment once the education program has been completed. However, sometimes such contractual agreements are referred to as golden handcuffs, illustrating that such financial security comes at a price.

The employer in such an arrangement is at a greater advantage to impose upon the clinician arrangements that he or she may find unattractive such as work hours, job description, and philosophy. If the clinician feels that entering into such an agreement is necessary to achieve the goals of higher education, negotiating the terms of employment simultaneously with the agreement for sponsorship helps to level the playing field a little. More discussion on contracts will occur in Chapter 6.

The clinician who finishes graduate school as a free agent must examine the employment possibilities or opportunities. The options available may include joining a practice of other healthcare providers, working for an agency or institution, or establishing a private practice.

Crisis: Access to Care

The clinician often is willing to practice in areas where recruitment and retention of physicians have been difficult. Because the costs of education, salaries, and liability insurance are lower, the clinician is a cost-effective solution to providing care to populations where reimbursement may be low or discounted.

When considering employment options, the clinician should evaluate what skills he or she possesses and determine if those skills are in demand. The clinician should evaluate whether there is a shortage of healthcare providers in the area or if there is a patient population that is underserved. Many clinicians' practices originated as a result of a lack of physician providers and/or the unmet demands of a defined patient population. Such crises within the healthcare system create opportunities for the disruptive innovator.

The healthcare crisis in the United States has been an employment avenue for healthcare providers that are educated sooner, command lower salaries, and are capable of caring for the majority of patients. In practices where the payor mix is largely indigent, the lower-cost provider can help offset lower payments or contractual allowances.

The savvy professional will do his or her homework when seeking em ployment. The clinician should be prepared to articulate to a board of directors or an administrator exactly how he or she can make a difference. The development of a business plan should begin with a description of who the clinician plans to serve, the needs of that population that are currently not being met, and how those needs can be met in a more efficient or cost-effective manner. The clinician should be prepared to answer the following questions:

- Are there shortages in the area?
- Are there practices that have recently closed?
- Is a group of providers near or at retirement?
- What is the average wait time to secure an appointment for a service?
- Is there an indigent population that is not being served or a significant number of people covered by a health plan with poor reimbursement?

After determining the need for services, the clinician should describe exactly how these needs can be met by the clinician and at what cost. A description of the education and experience of the clinician and how he or she can offer a solution to the problem should be discussed.

Crisis: The Internal Crisis

Another form of crisis that can present the provider with opportunities is the internal crisis. A personnel shortage may offer the provider with a temporary opportunity for additional work.

As a professional working within a system, the clinician should be vigilant for opportunities that enable the clinician to offer his or her services as a solution to a problem. Maternity leaves or other medical leaves of healthcare providers present an opportunity for a clinician to step in and assist in the interim. This benefits patients by alleviating long waits for appointments or the inconvenience of being overbooked on a full schedule. The practice receives much needed help, and the clinician has an opportunity to demonstrate skills, form alliances, and increase his or her value to an organization or practice.

A midwifery service offered to assist a local maternal-fetal medicine practice when two of their four physicians left to establish a practice in another state. The midwives were so well received by the patients that a full-time midwifery position was created within the service. In rural community hospitals where efforts to recruit physicians have failed, nurse-anesthetists have been hired to provide anesthesia services. Nurse-practitioners have been the foundations upon which many community health centers and clinics have been built.

In summary, healthcare crises such as geographic or demographic shortages can be a springboard or opportunity for the disruptive innovator. The rising cost of health care is a crisis that offers the opportunity for clinicians to establish an alternative model of care that offers cost-effective, satisfying health care to the general population without sacrificing quality. Disruptive innovators who specialize in risk assessment and health promotion within a system that allows for physician consultation, collaboration, and/or referral can offer a solution to the high cost of health care. Such a model would work collaboratively, not competitively, with traditional medicine.

The clinician should look for crises for which he or she can offer a solution. The disruptive innovator is ideally suited to intervene in situations that create problems in health care by converting a crisis into an opportunity.

NOTES

1. M. Breckinridge, *Wide Neighborhoods, A Story of the Frontier Nursing Service* (Lexington, KY: University Press of Kentucky, 1981).

2. American Association of Physician's Assistants, http://www.aapa.org (accessed 6/2003).

3. University of Kansas, SRIS Database, 20th Day Extract, Fall Semesters, 1990–1999.

4. Editorial, "Medical School Applications, A Disconcerting Drop," *American Medical News,* October 21, 2002, http://amednews.com (accessed 4/2003).

5. C. M. Christensen, R. Bohmer, and J. Kenagy, "Will Disruptive Innovations Cure Health Care?" *Harvard Business Review,* September–October 2000, 102–111.

CHAPTER 2

PLAYING BY THE RULES

It is said, "a rose is a rose," similarly, "a physician is a physician," thus making reciprocity for physicians as they move from one practice to another rather simple. The physician must apply for individual licensure in the state or country in which he or she plans to practice, but there is little dispute about the physician's scope of practice or authority. The physician also enjoys the privilege of insurance companies credentialing him or her without question, thus authorizing payment for services rendered, provided the physician fills out the proper forms and agrees to participate with the insurance plan.

For the clinician, the boundaries between states and practices are not so seamless. Rules and regulations differ from state to state and within local institutions. For the clinician to practice, he or she must gain a working understanding of the rules that define the legal scope of practice in the locale in which the clinician intends to work. Imagine a pyramid with each successive level becoming more detailed and specific as to the rights and privileges that are granted the clinician. This chapter will discuss each subset of rules that impact the clinician.

FEDERAL LAW

At the base of the pyramid is the federal government. The *Federal Register* is a document that is published weekly and contains information about proposed and adopted regulations or sections of the regulations. The *Federal Register* also contains comments, suggestions, and history regarding specific regulations. Most public libraries have copies of the *Federal Register*. The clinician should become familiar with the sections of the Medicaid and Medicare regulations that pertains to his or her specific category of provider.

The Center for Medicare and Medicaid Services (CMS), formally known as the Health Care Financing Administration (HCFA), revises, identifies, and implements the rules for compensation of services provided to enrollees in government programs. CMS determines the payment amount and under what conditions services provided by clinicians are reimbursed. Currently, clinicians are reimbursed at a reduced amount of the physician's fee schedule. To date, no data suggests that this rate of reimbursement is appropriate. It can be speculated that an ideal formula would include the amount of work effort required, the expense of providing a service, and the malpractice insurance costs of the clinician. Given such a formula, the discounted reimbursement would primarily reflect a difference in the cost of liability insurance because all other factors would remain equal.

STATE LAW

The clinician can obtain information about individual state licensing requirements by contacting the state board of licensing. Once an application for licensure is received by the licensing agency, it may take several weeks before the license is received by the clinician. Clinicians who anticipate working in a given state would be proactive by beginning the licensing process as soon as possible to avoid delays. Students awaiting graduation from a formal education program or awaiting certification from an accrediting organization should obtain the application for licensure prior to completing their education program or receiving results of the certifying exam, thus shortening the interval between certification and licensure.

Dual licensure is required in some states when licensure for an advanced practice nurse is sought. The clinician may be required to obtain licensure as a registered nurse as well as separate licensure for the specific field of advanced nurse practice. In this case, if the clinician intends to practice in a state where he or she has not been previously licensed as a registered nurse, the clinician may be wise to obtain licensure as a registered nurse before completing the graduate program. Many states allow nurses who have completed a specialty education program to work as graduates within that specialty while awaiting certification and/or state licensure, provided that the clinician is licensed by the state as a registered nurse. States also vary with regards to reciprocity for the licensing of registered nurses. If the clinician intends to practice in a state in which he or she is not already licensed, the nurse should contact the board of nursing to obtain information regarding licensure and begin that process while waiting to complete the graduate program or receive certification.

Individual states further define and describe the practice of the clinician. Three major categories are addressed in state rules and regulations: scope of practice, prescriptive authority, and relationship with the physician(s). The states also define the specifics of the Medicaid and State Children's Health Insurance Program (SCHIP) programs.

States vary as to where the rules and regulations are found concerning specific types of clinicians. Examples of regulatory bodies include the board of nursing, the board of public health, the midwifery board, and medical boards. An examination of the rules and regulations pertinent to practicing in any state is necessary to determine requirements for licensure. Educational preparation, sponsorship, certification, and other licensing prerequisites are as diverse as the states themselves. Within these regulations, the state also defines what healthcare services a clinician in the state is licensed to provide (scope of practice). The state may broadly define the clinician's scope of practice, leaving the actual details to individual practices and organizations, or it may define a specific scope of practice.

Prescriptive authority, whether independent or delegated, is defined in state rules and regulations. In some states, the clinician does not have the authority to write prescriptions. In others, the clinician may only write prescriptions for nonscheduled drugs. Some states delegate the writing of prescriptions to clinicians following preagreed upon formularies. In some cases, the state limits the number of clinicians a physician may supervise. Still others grant independent prescriptive authority to all healthcare providers. Many states granting prescriptive authority to clinicians require continuing education in order to maintain prescriptive privileges.

The relationship of the clinician to a physician or physicians is also described in individual state rules and regulations. Words such as *direction* or *supervision* are the nemesis of most clinicians. Even clinicians who do not, by law, possess independent licensure tend to resent the terms *supervision* or *direction* as it applies to their practice. One could interpret those terms as meaning clinicians are unable to think independently or lack the ability to exercise clinical judgment. The definition of such terms by local organizations or practices can restrict the scope of practice of the clinician at times beyond logic or reason. One could ask, "Of what value is the clinician, if the terms 'direction' or 'supervision' require physician presence or documentation that duplicates or replicates what the clinician has already done?" The original intent of such language was to ensure quality and safety in the delivery of health care. However, the terms now are weapons used in turf battles when traditional medicine is threatened by the practice of clinicians.

By definition, some clinicians are **independent practitioners**. The word *independent,* in this case, refers to licensure and does not in any way reject the interdependence all providers of a multidisciplinary healthcare team rely upon to provide comprehensive care to their patients. Other clinicians are not individually licensed and are thus dependent on physicians in order to practice.

Regardless of the language, a collaborative relationship should exist between each clinician and physician. This is not intended to tie the hands of the clinician, but allows for a formal mechanism of consultation, collaboration, and/or referral. When the clinician encounters a situation that he or she is not qualified to manage, care of the patient is expedited when a formal relationship exists between the clinician originally providing care to the patient and a professional prepared to render more-skilled care. Some states require such an agreement, written or verbal, in order to license or grant prescriptive authority to a clinician.

LOCAL RULES AND REGULATIONS

Hospitals, clinics, and other facilities or organizations describe and define the practice of clinicians in their **bylaws**. It would stand to reason that the bylaws of these organizations would reflect the current state law as it relates to the clinician; however, this is often *not* the case. Individual bylaws may not extend privileges to a clinician beyond that which is granted according to state rules and regulations; however, language that further restricts the clinician is common.

If the clinician is the first of his or her type to join an organization, an educational process should precede the development of such bylaws. The clinician is the individual who possesses the most comprehensive knowledge about the rules governing his or her practice, and thus it is logical that the clinician would be directly involved in the process. If the clinician plans to join an organization that is unfamiliar with his or her specific type of practice, the clinician should offer himself or herself as a resource to the organization. In preparation for this, the clinician should obtain information about state rules and regulations that assist in the definition of the specific practice. The clinician's professional organization at the state and national level can be of great assistance with this. However, the clinician should be cautious when negotiating, taking care to avoid acquiescing to points or language now that may be regretted later.

If the clinician anticipates obtaining hospital privileges, the clinician should examine and be familiar with the Joint Commission on Accreditation of Healthcare Organizations' (JCAHO) rules and regulations. All hospitals anticipating or maintaining JCAHO accreditation must follow rules for credentialing staff as defined by JCAHO. According to these rules, rights and privileges are often dependent on how the clinician is defined in the medical staff bylaws.

THE PHYSICIAN CONNECTION

The clinician's relationship with the collaborating physician should begin with honest and open conversations about scope of practice, collaborative agreements, and communication. To most clinicians, the physician is an ally, not the enemy.

Early in the process of forming a relationship with either an employer or a collaborating physician, collaborative agreements should be mutually developed. Collaborative or practice agreements describe the relationship between the clinician and the physician. They also describe the legal basis for practice and include guidelines for practice. Practice guidelines differ from protocols in that they are guidelines that allow for flexibility in practice, clinical judgment, and individualized care. Delegated prescriptive authority is usually addressed in the practice guidelines, as well as a formulary of approved drugs to be prescribed by the provider. A protocol can be viewed as a cookbook of recipes that does not allow for deviation, creativity, or personalization. Protocols may describe a procedure or policy from which one cannot deviate, for example, a protocol for inserting an intrauterine device.

Because practice guidelines help establish the legal basis for practice, copies of outdated or old guidelines should be archived because they will be consulted in case of litigation. As practice evolves, or as the clinician incorporates more skills into his or her clinical practice, the guidelines should be updated periodically.

The clinician, like all professionals, functions under a system of rules and regulations that govern and define the legal basis for practice. Often there is opportunity to aid in the development of these rules, in which case the provider should be prepared to offer educated, expert advice on the subject. It is much easier to write the rules correctly the first time than to cave in to pressure to not make waves and try to affect change later. Avoiding confrontation only delays the inevitable as the clinician strives to practice up to his or her potential and level of expertise.

As the clinician progresses through his or her education program, documentation that supports scope of practice should be collected in anticipation of participating in discussions related to scope of practice. The clinician should also begin to research the rules and regulations that will affect his or her practice. Being prepared and seeking guidance from seasoned colleagues will facilitate a smooth transition from student to licensed provider. Relocating to another state, practice, or organization may also require the clinician to investigate and then articulate the *rules* regarding his or her legal basis for practice. Maintaining a file that contains pertinent documents that can be used in such situations can help streamline this process.

CHAPTER 3

NO TAXATION WITHOUT REPRESENTATION

The previous chapter discussed the importance of understanding the rules and regulations governing practice. Each clinician should be familiar with the specific regulations pertaining to his or her professional practice within the state he or she wishes to practice. As pointed out in Chapter 2, laws and/or regulations that help to define the clinician's legal basis for practice exist on many levels. This chapter will discuss the importance of rule development as it pertains to the involvement of the clinician.

Hospital administrators, physicians, and office managers can all be equally ignorant as to the legal basis for practice of the clinician. Without guidance, guidelines or bylaws can be developed that severely restrict practice or actually place the physician or clinician at increased risk for liability. Although the idea of approaching the hospital credentials committee or medical board gives many clinicians a good set of nervous jitters, it is a necessary evil if one is to enjoy the rights and privileges for which one is qualified.

As the title of this chapter suggests, the clinician should attempt to participate in rule development as it occurs on a variety of levels. Without the guidance and input of the clinician, rules may be developed out of ignorance that may unnecessarily restrict the practice of the clinician. Although most clinicians loath the thought of attending meetings, failure to be present and represent the profession may result in restrictions or prohibitions that could have been avoided had the clinician taken the time to attend.

When the clinician does attend, the clinician has a responsibility to the profession he or she represents to maintain a noticeable and productive presence at meetings, committees, or social gatherings. Not only must the clinician have a presence, the clinician must also have a voice. It does not serve the profession if the clinician merely sits at the table, but never makes a contribution. The wise clinician will observe the environment and assess the personalities of those present to determine how and when it is best to contribute to a meeting.

When the clinician is representing himself or herself or the profession as a whole, the clinician should come to meetings prepared with documentation that supports his or her position on the topics to be discussed, especially if controversy is expected. The clinician should anticipate all arguments and be prepared to logically and legally defend his or her position. Emotion never has a place in these discussions. A tirade or other theatrical display destroys the professional atmosphere of the meeting and the message is lost in the delivery.

This chapter will discuss professional involvement that should exist on various levels to ensure that there is no taxation without representation, or stated another way: Policy is not created that affects the clinician without benefit of the clinician's input.

LEGISLATION

In Chapter 9, the clinician is advised to develop a sense of political awareness and to get and remain politically active with the help of local and national organizations.

BYLAWS

Organizations large and small operate under a set of rules as defined in their *bylaws.* Bylaws differ from organization to organization, but most generally include rules of procedure and policy. For the clinician, medical staff bylaws in organizations such as hospitals define administrative and clinical procedures as they apply to care delivery within the organization. The bylaws describe the rights and privileges granted to those who provide care within the hospital and address issues such as clinical privileges, quality management, medical records documentation, and discipline.

When a clinician joins an organization or seeks privileges within a hospital, the bylaws must be revised to specifically address the function of the clinician within the organization. The clinician may work in an environment in which all of the rules were established prior to his or her arrival. In some cases, without the input of the clinician or others in the same profession, the rules may not accurately reflect the clinician's legal scope of practice. Although hospital bylaws often are in concert with state laws, such is not always the case. This may be due to inaccurate information about state laws pertaining to the clinician's practice or a deliberate choice by the hospital to restrict the clinician's practice beyond state laws. To prevent such situations, the clinician should assertively insist on participating on committees charged with developing policy changes or bylaws. If the clinician complacently or naively waits for bylaws to be written by others, he or she may not like the results. It takes more work to revise an unfriendly set of bylaws than to construct them properly in the first place.

When contemplating the construction of medical staff bylaws that will describe privileges, voting rights, and peer review practices of the clinician, the clinician should refer to and become familiar with the rules and regulations as defined by JCAHO. Hospitals accredited by JCAHO must comply with JCAHO rules regarding medical staff bylaws. JCAHO rules are updated periodically. Information may be obtained by accessing their Web site at http://www.jcaho.com.

COMMITTEES AND DEPARTMENT MEETINGS

Serving on hospital committees is often a function of members of the medical staff. The clinician is no exception. The clinician should ensure a place on peer review, quality control, or other pertinent committees. Disciplinary action or investigation on issues of quality should not be left to the domain of the physician. In most cases, the physician is not qualified to evaluate non-physician practice. Granted, standards of care are standards of care, but the clinician often approaches care from a different direction than a physician, thus it is critical for the clinician to insist on a seat on these committees.

Attendance at medical staff meetings, department meetings, or other gatherings illustrative of the hierarchy of organized medicine is one of the necessary evils when one is to be considered a professional. If a clinician is consistently absent at such meetings, decisions may be made that are contradictory to the practice of the clinician. Furthermore, the clinician's absence may send a message that he or she is not on the same level as others in the profession or perhaps cannot or will not be a valuable contributor to such discussions. This type of reticence may lead to misunderstandings, resentment, or hard feelings. Through such behavior, the clinician affirms that he or she is only a physician "extender" and grants, by his or her absence, the physician ultimate dominion and decision making with regards to the clinician's practice. Conversely, the presence of the clinician at such functions, both business and social, may give the appearance that the clinician is a professional member of the healthcare team with a voice and a vote. To be viewed as a valuable, respected, and intelligent professional, one must act like one. This includes attendance at functions and meetings.

PRACTICE GUIDELINES

Just as organizational bylaws define medical staff rules and regulations, practice agreements, or practice guidelines (the two terms are used interchangeably), describe how the clinician functions within his or her own practice. Practice agreements define the scope of practice of the clinician, define the legal basis for practice, and define the physician-clinician relationship. Practice agreements are not to be confused with protocols, which do not allow for clinical judgment or individualized care. Guidelines, instead, provide a framework for practice. The clinician should be the lead author of the practice agreements.

Writing practice guidelines, which can be a lengthy and tedious process, is another necessary evil to establish good practice. When the clinician writes the practice guidelines, he or she is intimately aware of what information is contained within them and feels a commitment to following them. The local or national organizations representing the clinician can be of valuable assistance when writing practice guidelines.

PRACTICE MEETINGS

The professional clinician must take care to participate in practice operations with as much due diligence as he or she gives to participation in a hospital or other organization's meetings and committees. Practice meetings are usually scheduled to address operational issues, changes, financial affairs, or clinical issues. By failing to attend or participate in these meetings, the clinician forfeits the right to provide feedback and make suggestions on how the practice runs. Some clinicians feel that they are entitled compensation for attending such meetings and are resentful when they occur after regular office hours. However, the rationale for scheduling meetings this way is to avoid disrupting patient schedules. If meetings occur during regular hours, the support staff is being paid and no revenue is being generated. Participation in practice meetings is an expectation of professionals and demonstrates a commitment to the practice. Failure to regularly attend practice meetings or to expect compensation for doing so is evidence of adopting a nonprofessional attitude and is not representative of professional behavior.

PROFESSIONAL ORGANIZATIONS

Local professional groups or chapters may influence practice on the local level. In order to assure that the interests of the clinician are represented, personal involvement in these groups is mandatory. Each state has professional organizations, including the medical society for physicians. The clinician has the option to serve as a consultant on committees within the medical society whose clinical interests are pertinent to the practice of the clinician. Again, the clinician is advised to play this role only if he or she is willing to speak up when appropriate.

SPECIAL INTEREST GROUPS

The clinician should also be a member of other committees within a practice, organization, or social structure that may make decisions that can impact the practice of the clinician. For instance, a local medical society or network may greatly influence practice within a certain locale. The clinician should also be familiar with patient support groups or societies whose members are clients or potential clients of the clinician.

Healthcare professionals are not by nature wallflowers or shrinking violets. The responsibility they assume by accepting innovative roles in health care should not end with the clinical care of patients. The clinician has many opportunities to represent his or her profession. Failure to do so not only reflects poorly on the professionalism of the clinician, but can have a costly impact on the clinician's practice. There may be times when the clinician must be assertive and insist on being included on committees or meetings that directly impact the clinician's practice. By exhibiting professional behavior and making valuable contributions, the clinician can assure his place and avoid taxation without representation.

CHAPTER 4

WHAT'S IN A NAME?

By now, many readers, if they have read the previous chapters, have bristled or taken offense at one or more of the variety of terms used in reference to the clinicians for whom this book was written. There is no universal term that compliments all types of healthcare providers who are not physicians. In fact, the most commonly used terms suggest such prejudice as to shed negative light on the clinicians themselves. Using the most accurate label, such as pediatric nurse-practitioner, physician's assistant, or nurse-midwife, may be the most accurate way to refer to a clinician, however, such practice is cumbersome when authoring a book. This chapter examines the various labels applied to clinicians.

Healthcare providers come in many packages with a multitude of labels, and the average consumer is ill equipped to discern among them with a high degree of accuracy. Further, without advanced preparation, concepts such as educational preparation, licensure, scope of practice, and qualifications of various members of the healthcare team are lost as well. This is not surprising given the variety of clinicians in, and complexity of, today's healthcare delivery system. Combine that with differences in state and local rules and regulations, and it is easy to see why the general public cannot tell the difference between a physician's assistant and a nurse-practitioner.

Physicians enjoy a great deal of state-to-state reciprocity with respect to education, licensure, and scope of practice. Insurance companies and hospitals generally agree on the process for credentialing and extending privileges to physicians. Programs such as quality management and peer review have long been the purview of physicians. Likewise, consumers are not at all unclear as to the role of the physician.

When the ignorance of consumers is combined with that of legislators, administrators, insurance companies, and physicians themselves, the disruptive innovator has a high probability of being continuously misunderstood.

The language that has labeled nonphysician providers has been anything but flattering.

NONPHYSICIAN PROVIDER

Consider the term **nonphysician provider**. It describes what the clinician *is not* more than what he or she *is*. The term does nothing to define the unique skills and training possessed by the clinician, nor does it give the consumer any idea about the specialty area of health care in which the clinician is proficient. The term nonphysician provider categorically labels the clinician as something less than the accepted standard of care.

MIDLEVEL PROVIDER

Similarly, another term, **midlevel provider**, has been used to label nonphysician clinicians. This term suggests a level of care that is something less than the best. The term *mid*level also implies half the education, training, or quality of a physician. Are we to conclude then that registered nurses, medical assistants, and such are *low*-level providers?

PHYSICIAN EXTENDER

Another descriptive term applied to clinicians is **physician extender**. This is a well-intentioned term because it implies that the clinician extends the practice of the physician. It was perhaps this term that attracted physicians to the concept of incorporating nurse-midwives, nurse-practitioners, physician's assistants, and clinical nurse specialists into their practices. By employing an "extender," it was argued that the physician could decrease wait time for appointments, thus improving access to care. Physicians were also enamored with the argument that the physician could bill for the services provided by the extender while providing services simultaneously themselves. This served to double the productivity of the physician without doubling overhead costs—quite a convincing argument.

Although the term extender seems somewhat logical when taken in this context, it again fails to credit the clinician with critical thinking, clinical judgment, or responsibility independent of the physician. Barriers to practice are imposed because the extender is expected to be linked with a physician. This creates problems with licensure and regulations because the words *supervision* and *direction* appear in language describing the legal basis for practice. Billing for services independently is problematic and often impossible because insurance companies do not have mechanisms to credential the nonphysician, instead linking the clinician with the "supervising" physician.

Public health information about the volume of patients cared for by nonphysicians is often inaccurate because much of this information is gleaned from billing records. If bills are generated by the physician, the statistics do not account for work done by the nonphysician provider. Thinking of a clinician as an extender only continues to propagate the myth that the clinician is merely an extension of a physician.

PARAPROFESSIONAL

Another term used to describe the nonphysician clinician is the term **paraprofessional**. The prefix *para* means "beside" or "an accessory to." This term has been applied to legal assistants, teacher's aides, and others whose specific responsibility is to assist the professional with their workload. Such positions bear very little responsibility, and their function is dependent on the professional for whom they work. The term paraprofessional infers that the nonphysician healthcare provider is more technical than professional. Nothing could be further from the truth. Nonphysician providers possess technical clinical skills, but use those skills based on individual assessment and the employment of clinical judgment, reasoning, and problem solving.

ADVANCED PRACTICE (REGISTERED) NURSE

The term **advanced practice nurse** (**APN**) or **advanced practice registered nurse** (**APRN**) commonly refers to nurses who have taken on additional roles and or responsibilities, thereby expanding their scope of nursing practice. This may be achieved through postgraduate education, internships, or certification programs. The term signifies that the clinician possesses a basic nursing degree but lumps together all nurses with some form of additional education.

Nurse practitioners vary greatly in their areas of clinical expertise. Yet, a certified nurse-midwife whose educational history also includes a basic nursing education is licensed and credentialed differently than a nurse-practitioner. The term APN or APRN also excludes other nonphysician providers such as the physician's assistant.

ALLIED HEALTHCARE PROVIDER

Perhaps the term that most accurately describes the nonphysician provider is the term **allied healthcare provider**. *Merriam-Webster* defines *allied* as "having or being in close association" or "connected." Because nonphysician clinicians often feel like square pegs in traditional medicine's round holes, a connective title should not be viewed as undesirable.

EAST OR WEST, WHICH IS BEST?

The terms presented in this chapter illustrate how difficult it is to name a group of clinicians that are not physicians with a term that does not undermine their education, expertise, and autonomy. Because respective areas of practice vary greatly, clinicians should call themselves precisely what they are whenever possible. This avoids interpersonal misunderstandings and confusion. For example, a pediatric nurse-practitioner differs in scope of practice from a women's health nurse-practitioner.

If more than one type of clinician exists within the same organization, attempts to label them both with the same term will ultimately result in the misrepresentation of one or more clinicians. Organizations often lump together all nonphysician providers when addressing issues of productivity and contracting. Should the nurse-midwives who cover deliveries 7 days a week be held as a benchmark for the physician's assistants who never work evenings, weekends, or holidays? Should the nurse-practitioner in practice A who triages all of the after-hours phone calls, makes hospital rounds, and performs inpatient histories and physicals be compensated the same as the nurse-practitioner in practice B who does only clinical research?

For these reasons, clinicians should resist attempts to be labeled by one generic term, especially in instances where the only common denominator is the fact that they are not physicians.

Labels and names differ, much like clinicians' credentials. The initials behind one's name often do not clearly define the clinician's role, degree, or licensure. When working within a healthcare system, the clinician should take care to ensure that the initials or credentials he or she possesses are unique to his or her practice. For example, imagine the confusion that arises when Certified Nurse-Midwives (CNMs) practice in the same organization that calls its charge nurses clinical nurse managers (CNMs).

Conversely, there may be times when a duplication of terms is justified. A term commonly used in a management hierarchy is the term *director*. The American College of Nurse-Midwives commonly identifies a lead midwife in a practice as a service director. Conflicts may arise in an institution where the term *director* denotes certain privileges or responsibilities that the organization does not extend to the nurse-midwife or the midwife may simply fit into another management structure within the same organization. Yet, because the term *service director* is a term recognized on a national level within the profession, the nurse-midwife should have the right to bear the title director within such an organization.

While some may feel discussions about names may be fruitless or a useless expenditure of energy, others may get passionate about the use or abuse of terms applied to healthcare providers. Whether or not this is a battle the clinician is willing to fight, when the opportunity arises to affix a name, clinicians should choose one that most closely represents the clinical practice performed.

CHAPTER 5

FRIEND OR FOE, WHO YOU SHOULD KNOW

Anyone entering the world of business, no matter the profession, should contemplate how he or she will interact with others and determine key individuals or groups that should be contacted. It is good business to market oneself to others in both the lay and healthcare community, but it is particularly important to the clinician whose complete role may not be understood clearly by the general population. This chapter discusses some ideas and recommendations for engaging in public relations. **Public relations** differs from **marketing** in that marketing is done to sell a product or service, whereas public relations promotes an understanding or acceptance of a person or persons.

MAKE A GOOD FIRST IMPRESSION

Logically, the clinician has only one opportunity to make a first impression, therefore it should be a good one. When interviewing for a position or when introducing oneself, it is important to look, and to act, like a professional. Regardless of one's substance, perception is reality, and people are judged by appearances. It is important to avoid playing into stereotypes and misperceptions by assuming a universally professional appearance.

Open-toed shoes without stockings are forbidden, even after an expensive pedicure. With regards to nails, no clinician should sport one-inch acrylics! Trendy clothing and jewelry should be avoided; leave the uterus earrings at home. Hair, beards, and mustaches should be neat. As a simple rule, clothing that is one step above what one would normally wear to work should be worn.

This advice may seem to some as unnecessarily stating the obvious, however, many administrators have reported a general state of disrepair among recent applicants. Do not take chances. When in doubt, err toward the conservative. Similarly, when a meeting with the organization's board or other community leaders, take the power suit out of mothballs even if your typical work wear may be dress casual.

Demeanor is also important when presenting oneself to the community or organizational leadership. Make eye contact, avoid the use of slang and, by all means, practice a firm handshake. Prepare and rehearse presentations, making sure to adhere to any time constraints. Do the due diligence and know the audience, whether they number in the hundreds or just one.

When interviewing, be prepared to ask questions as well as answer them. This demonstrates interest in the practice or organization and sheds light on your investigative and reasoning skills. Above all, relax and be yourself. Though you've likely submitted one in advance, bring a copy of your resume or curriculum vitae.

A resume is a brief account of one's academic and professional experience. A curriculum vitae, or CV (the terms are often used synonymously), is more frequently used by professionals and includes professional memberships, honors and awards, publications, and research completed by the applicant. Whether a CV or resume, be sure the document is of good quality. Do not embellish any information, remain factual.

ADMINISTRATORS, BOARD MEMBERS, AND OFFICE MANAGERS, OH MY!

Do not assume that others in the practice clearly understand your intended role. Even the administrator responsible for interviewing or hiring may not fully understand your scope of practice or the regulations that affect it. If you are the first of your specialty to enter an organization, a formal presentation to the board or administrative team should be considered.

Such a presentation should include information about federal and state rules and regulations as well as a description of your education and scope of practice. If appropriate, you should describe the target patient population you hope to serve and additional ways you can be of value to the practice or organization. Prepare a packet that includes documents that support the information you present such as the state's rules and regulations; JCAHO rules; local demographics, if applicable; and professional literature produced by national organizations that represent your specialty.

Do not stop with administrators. The educational process should trickle down through each layer of the organization. Department heads of the laboratory, pharmacy, nutrition services, and radiology departments need to become acquainted with you and develop an understanding about your role within the organization. People will find it much harder to construct barriers to your practice when they connect a name to a friendly face. If all orders or requisitions come in the name of the physician in the practice, you become an invisible entity within the organization if you have failed to make contact with other professionals. This advice also holds true for clinicians who are not a part of an organization. In addition, you should formally introduce yourself to local leaders of businesses that may support your practice.

PUBLIC RELATIONS

Another department head worthy of your attention is the public relations director. Spend time discussing with this person what you do and the healthcare areas in which you are especially interested. Offer yourself as a resource when the organization is approached by the media regarding current trends in health care that fall within your area of expertise. Volunteer to write an article for the organization's newsletter or the local newspaper.

The public relations department maintains a list of people willing to represent the organization on various topics. Even if you shudder at the thought of looking into a television camera, there are many other opportunities to interact with the media such as radio, newspaper, or phone interviews.

Contact the health editor of the local newspaper. Discuss areas of special interest and topics in which you may be considered an expert. Submit or collaborate on an article that introduces you and your practice to the community. For example, if you are the first nurse-midwife to practice in the area, write an article about midwifery.

A word of caution: If you are employed by an organization, there may be rules of procedure to follow when contacting, or being contacted by, the media. Discuss this process when meeting with the public relations director. If there is a topic that you wish to address or if you have a story that may be of interest to the public, the public relations director can assist you with contacting the media to share your story.

If you are not a part of an organization, it is still very important to remain on the look out for topics that may be of interest to others that enable you to get media attention and subsequently market your practice.

SUPPORT STAFF

Do not limit your interpersonal public relations campaign to department heads and administrators. Nor should you underestimate the value of getting to know the housekeeping and maintenance staff. Remember that most healthcare providers rely heavily on word of mouth for their advertising. Everyone with whom you come in contact is a potential new patient. Additionally, unless you want to clean or maintain your own work environment, allocate some time to befriending your support staff.

Consider spending a fair amount of time with clerical staff and the billing department. The intake person in a practice needs to be familiar with what types of patients you are qualified to see and any associated restrictions or requirements. Discuss the time you will need to see each type of patient so that a scheduling template can be developed to meet individual patient needs and to ensure a reasonable measure of productivity.

It is not unusual for billing staff to feel that billing for anyone other than a physician is illegal and may land them in jail for committing fraud. Even worse, some might believe that billing under a physician for a service provided by someone else smacks of deception! Because the viability of a clinician within a practice or organization is directly related to the ability to produce revenue, it is advantageous to see that clinical activity is accurately accounted for and compensation is obtained.

Expecting the billing department to be well versed in the payment nuances for professionals other than physicians is a dangerous assumption when one's career is at stake. The clinician can enlist the aide of national organizations representing his or her specialty area to determine billing rules and regulations specific to the state of practice. See Chapter 13 for more information on billing rules and regulations.

PHYSICIANS

Public relations begins, but does not end, in the workplace. The healthcare provider should find opportunities to socialize with other medical professionals, especially physicians, at such functions as medical staff dinners, foundation fundraisers, and country club luncheons. Although donning tuxedo or evening gown may not be the forte of the clinician, stepping out into the medical community at social functions provides the opportunity to rub elbows with other members of the healthcare community. It is much easier and less threatening to discuss one's vocation at a cocktail party than at a lectern or in a board room. Attendance at such functions also confirms the clinician's status as a healthcare *professional.* So, break out the golf clubs!

NURSES

Two of the most important and influential groups of people that any clinician must befriend are the nurses and medical assistants. Not only do nurses comprise a commanding proportion of the healthcare team, they are in a unique position to influence and educate large numbers of people. Make no mistake, in a healthcare setting, physicians may hold the prestige, but nurses wield the power.

Nurses may originally be skeptical of the qualifications and roles of nonphysician providers. Some nurses are threatened by the presence of the nonphysician provider with respect to authority. They may be anxious that the nonphysician provider will replace or displace them. Some view other providers as an additional layer between them and the physician. Because nurses are strong patient advocates by nature, they will need reassurance that their patients will be receiving care that is of the highest quality.

Once the clinician is able to win the trust and respect of the nursing staff, he or she will have strong advocates within the organization. The clinician should plan to attend formal and informal meetings with nursing staff to discuss the role of the nonphysician provider and how this role will interface with theirs.

THE HEALTHCARE COMMUNITY

The clinician should look for opportunities to serve on professional committees or task forces. Participating in such activities affords the clinician with the opportunity to interact with others in the healthcare community and to educate them about the clinician's particular practice. Forming such liaisons will make up the infrastructure of the clinician's professional peer group.

By joining local special interest groups such as the March of Dimes or American Cancer Society, you can contribute to the work of these societies as well as increase your exposure. Offer to do speaking engagements at schools, senior centers, community centers, societies, churches, or clubs. These organizations commonly offer local events that provide a venue for educating the public, as well as community leaders, about the role of the clinician.

THE BUSINESS COMMUNITY

The clinician opening his or her own practice should endeavor to form relationships with other community leaders. An easy first step is to join the local chamber of commerce. This provides the opportunity to market one's business as well as to interact with other businesspeople in the community. As a member of the chamber of commerce, the clinician should be sure that his or her practice is included in local publications that introduce residents to local businesses.

The clinician can also look for opportunities to serve on committees or programs within the community that allow for opportunities to interact with other community leaders. Membership in local charities or special interest groups may be an avenue for marketing. The clinician can offer to sponsor a local theater group or advertise in a school athletic program. All of these ways help to expand the clinician's exposure beyond the healthcare community and into the business community.

EDUCATION PROGRAMS

Schedule a meeting with the directors of clinical education programs in the area. The clinician can offer to guest lecture for nursing programs or other forums for higher education. Students of advanced practice programs are also in need of clinical sites in which to perform the hands-on portion of their education. The clinician may offer to serve as a preceptor in these programs. If a medical school is nearby, offer to lecture or serve as a clinical preceptor for its program. The return on the investment of working with medical students is worth the extra time it takes to supervise them. They are the future medical staff members that will have the ability to influence policy, bylaws revisions, and credentialing of nonphysician providers. By gaining their respect and appreciation for the competency and role of the nonphysician members of the health care team, goodwill can be engendered toward future clinicians. Do not miss the opportunity to discuss with them the education and expertise of the clinician so that they develop a rudimentary understanding about your profession.

VOLUNTEER

The clinician should participate, whenever possible, in volunteer activities that generate exposure to the community. Staff a booth at a health fair or career expo. Serve a community organization such as a crisis pregnancy center, blood pressure screening clinic, immunization clinic, or free clinic. Seek out the athletic directors of area schools and offer to do sports physicals. Make sure you always take along a stack of business cards and brochures that describe your practice and/or profession.

Many large organizations require that their employees participate in health education programs. The clinician may be able to provide some of this education, thus gaining exposure to another group of people and an employer or company.

Similarly, contact local ambulance companies and offer to lecture to paramedics or emergency medical technicians for either their basic or continuing education programs.

SALES REPRESENTATIVES

The clinician should also try to take the time to meet with representatives of drug companies when they call on the practice. Drug reps, as they are commonly called, supply the clinician with samples and a wealth of information on advances in research and practice. Drug reps also are usually up to date on current information in the lay literature and may assist the clinician in finding information commonly sought by patients. However, the clinician should be cautioned that although drug representatives provide a wealth of new information, they are in fact salespeople who are primarily interested in promoting their product.

POLITICIANS

Lastly, the clinician should make time to contact area policy makers. Follow politics with enough interest to know when legislation is contemplated that may affect your practice. Offer yourself as the resident expert in your clinical field and make yourself available as a resource to legislators and their aides. Schedule an appointment to introduce yourself and your profession. Assume that the legislator knows nothing about your field of practice and has only 10 minutes to learn about it. See Chapter 9 for more discussion about legislators.

PATIENTS

There is no stronger advocate or marketing tool than the satisfied patient, yet many clinicians overlook this abundant resource. Studies have shown that recommendations from family or friends account for a large proportion of a practice's referrals. The clinician should give his or her patients permission to make those referrals. Have business cards at the check-out counter and invite patients to take them to give to their friends. When a new patient gives the name of an established patient as the source of their interest in the practice, the clinician may take a moment to send a note of thanks or call the patient to express appreciation for the referral. Such personal attention to marketing reaps many rewards for the clinician laboring to grow a thriving practice.

It is often who a clinician knows that may give him or her the advantage of practicing in a friendly, supportive environment. While politicking and socializing may be out of the comfort zone of many clinicians, introducing oneself to various leaders in both the lay and professional community may dispel some of the bias and ignorance that negatively influences or restricts the ability of the clinician to practice.

CHAPTER 6

SIGNING ON THE DOTTED LINE

Edward J. Annen, Jr.
Attorney at Law

The most important aspect of your relationship with either your employer or with a private practice for which you are providing services is your contract. You might have reached all sorts of verbal understandings, but if you enter into a written contract, those verbal understandings, except in very limited circumstances, are of no value. (Most states will permit testimony as to verbal understandings and discussions when there is a written contract, only for the purposes of assisting the court in determining the intent of a part of a written contract that is not clear on its face.) This chapter will explore how to approach and analyze your contract.

It is important to understand that what your employer will insist be in the contract or what terms the employer is willing to consider changing as an inducement to have you sign the contract is largely dependent on the particular labor market for your position. If there are 50 applicants for 2 positions, you most likely will be presented with a boilerplate contract containing language favorable to the employer, with the employer unwilling to change any of that language. However, if you are one of 10 applicants for 50 positions, generally your employer will consider changing aspects of the contract to induce you to become an employee. The labor market often drives the nature of a contract.

SPECIFICS OF A CONTRACT

A contract generally specifies the following:

- The parties to the contract
- The consideration supporting the contract (consideration can be wages, salary, earnings, and mutual promises)
- The duration of the contract
- The rights and obligations of each party entering into the contract

- The rights and obligations of each party in the event one of the parties breaches or breaks the contract

EMPLOYEE HANDBOOKS

During the past decade, employee handbooks (or manuals) have come into extensive use. Most generally, they integrate with your actual contract, and in most cases they are deemed to be a part of the contract. An employee handbook will not usually address the components of a contract, but will likely deal with issues such as dress codes, benefits, vacation days, personal days, disciplinary matters, and so on. It is very important that when you examine a contract you also examine and review prior to signing the contract any employee handbook that accompanies it.

LEGAL CONSIDERATIONS

First and foremost, before you sign a contract, you should consult with a lawyer. Tell that lawyer what you believe you are contracting to do and what your expectations are. Show the lawyer the contract and any employee handbook *prior to signing it.* Most people do not bring their employment contract or handbook to a lawyer until after the contract is signed and a dispute arises. Generally, you can expect to pay very modest legal fees to have the lawyer review the contract and handbook with you and highlight special points of legal significance. What are those points?

- Does your contract describe you as an *employee at will,* or are you employed for a term of weeks, months, or years? An employee at will can be discharged at anytime for no cause at all. (However, regardless of whether you are an at will employee, you still cannot be discharged for discriminatory reasons. The law protects you from being discharged because of your race, color, national origin, or sex. Each state sets forth in their laws what constitutes discrimination in employment.) You may have verbally understood in May that you would be working until September, but, if you are an at will employee, you can be discharged in June and have no claim for lost income for the months of July and August.
- Does your contract term you an *employee* or an *independent contractor*? Generally, the law deems a person to be an independent contractor if they are so termed to be that in a contract and if they primarily provide their own working implements and provide their own direction, which is to say that they do not receive directions from a supervisor. This becomes important because if you are an independent contractor, the person you have contracted with does not have to withhold taxes, FICA, and so on, nor does the entity have to provide you benefits. It also is important because if you are an independent contractor, whatever liability (mal-

practice) or other insurance protections the entity you are contracting with has most probably will not apply to protect you. So if you are an independent contractor, make sure that your contract clearly spells out the insurance responsibilities of each party.

- If you are an independent contractor or otherwise contracting to provide services to an entity in a capacity other than that of employee, you need to have a clear written statement as to how billing rights are to be handled. Are you assigning your billing rights to the entity to collect the bills for you? If so, what obligation do they have to collect delinquent bills? How does bill collection affect your own compensation? It is advisable that all these issues be clearly addressed in the written contract.
- Make sure your contract clearly spells out the benefits you are to receive, if any, and under what circumstances those benefits can be taken away or modified.
- Clarify whether your contract references an employee handbook or employee manual, and if so, have a clear written understanding in the contract whether what is printed in the handbook or manual is part of the contract. As just one example, your employment contract may not say that you have to wear a white jacket to work. Your handbook or manual may declare that you do have to wear a white jacket to work. You need a clear written understanding as to whether a violation of what is in the handbook or manual constitutes a violation of the contract.
- Determine if your contract sets forth steps that are to be followed to resolve a dispute between the contracting parties. Again, this may require referencing a handbook or manual and determining how that document integrates with your contract. On numerous occasions over the years, employees present themselves to a lawyer after they have been discharged, basically saying, "It only happened one time, how can they fire me without giving a warning first. Is that legal?" My answer is always, "It may be legal or it may not be legal. Let me look at your contract and your employee handbook." More often than not, I have to show the person asking the question the language that says "You may be discharged without warning for any violation of this contract and the accompanying employee handbook."
- If you do have an employee handbook or manual, have the contract state in writing that you will be promptly notified of any changes to the handbook that may occur after you become employed, and that unless any changes are presented to you within a certain time frame they will not apply to you.
- Have the contract clearly state what you are allowed in terms of sick days, personal days, and vacation time. You may think it perfectly okay to take a day off of work with or without pay to attend Aunt Edna's funeral. Your contract and/or employee handbook may state something all together different.

- Finally, examine the contract closely as to what it sets forth as to remedies for a breach of the contract and where that breach is to be addressed. For example: Does your contract say that regardless of the term of the contract, if the employee is discharged he or she will receive only 2 weeks pay? Is your employer a national company? Does your contract state that "the forum for any breach of this contract is a court for a county in the state of Alaska" when your particular branch is in the state of Georgia? Do you want or can you afford to litigate a breach of your contract in a forum several thousands of miles away?

NONCOMPETITION CLAUSES

Other issues that may arise concerning an employment contract are **noncompetition clauses** and agreements. Most states now permit noncompetition clauses. States vary as to what such a clause must say and what is reasonable. Generally, noncompetition agreements require separate consideration. This is to say that a well-drafted noncompetition agreement/clause will state words to the effect of: "In addition to, and not as a part of the employee's earnings, employer tenders to employee $X.XX dollars to enter into this noncompetition agreement/clause."

You need to determine with your attorney what your state's requirements are, but most states require that the agreement be based upon an employer's reasonable competitive business interests. This involves questions of who are the competitors of your employer and where are they located? As an employee, are you privy to confidential information that enables your employer to more effectively compete against another entity? Is that information portable, which is to say could you successfully implement it with another entity? Generally, the greater your responsibility and the more firmly you are entrenched in a supervisory capacity, the more likely it is that your employer can show the need to protect a reasonable competitive business interest in requiring you to sign a noncompetition agreement.

In addition, most states require that a noncompetition agreement be reasonable as to its duration, geographical area, and type of employment or line of business. There are cases wherein a national company, such as an automobile manufacturer, has successfully enforced a nationwide noncompete against a senior vice president with all sorts of inside information as to advertising strategy, pricing strategy, and so on. But such situations are very rare, and the reasoning behind such rulings are generally not applicable to the healthcare field. Usually, a radius of 50 miles and a duration of 2 years is deemed reasonable. But again, this can vary widely and may depend on the unique circumstances covering your field and your geographic area. It is unlikely that your employer, through a noncompete agreement, could successfully prevent you from being employed by a similar entity several states away. It is also unlikely that your employer could successfully prevent you from being employed by a competing entity for a period of 20 years. The courts apply rules of reason in enforcing noncompetition agreements. For example, if you are privy to confidential advertising and pricing information in your field that has enabled your employer to successfully compete with a competing entity 20 miles away, it is likely a court would enforce your non-competition agreement and prevent you from being employed by that competing entity for a period of a few years.

OWNERSHIP INTEREST

Finally, depending on your particular circumstances, another aspect of an employment contract may spell out the terms under which you can eventually become a shareholder, partner, or limited liability company member, depending on the specific entity employing you. If you are entering into a contractual relationship wherein you will expect in the future to obtain an ownership interest, you need to ensure that the contract clarifies the following:

- Under what conditions and/or time duration will an ownership interest be made available to you?
- What is the nature of that ownership interest; that is, are you a partner, shareholder, or member?
- Will there be a buy-in requirement to obtain ownership? Will you be expected to tender funds for stock, or a partner's interest, or a member's interest? If so, how much?
- What will be your return on your ownership interest? Will you receive a percentage of profits and be responsible for a percentage of loss corresponding to your percentage of ownership?
- Under what conditions can you be required to relinquish your ownership interest and under what financial conditions?
- You should ask to see the governing document of the business entity in which you would be obtaining an ownership interest, that is to say the articles of incorporation and by-laws if a closely held corporation, the partnership agreement if a partnership, or the articles of organization and members' agreement if a limited liability company.
- You also need to know what happens to your ownership interest in the event of your death or permanent disability.

The purpose of this chapter is to convey to you the legal significance of employment contracts and to prevent you from just aimlessly signing on the dotted line. You must truly know and understand what you are contracting to do and to have done for you.

One final note: This chapter largely presumes that you will not be a union employee. If in fact your employee category is a unionized position, the vast majority of what is in this chapter will not apply to you. This is primarily because most of the items addressed in this chapter will be addressed in the labor agreement bargained for and entered into between the employer and employees' union. At a minimum, however, you should ask to see a copy of that bargaining agreement so that you know what rights you have as a union employee. The most basic of these rights would be bumping rights—the right to bump into another's job if you are senior in tenure to a similar employee category with less tenure, and so on.

CHAPTER 7

MANAGING LIABILITY

One of the harsh realities of providing health care is medical liability. The clinician must be realistic and understand that we live in a litigious society and that medical malpractice is a potential threat to all healthcare providers. This chapter will discuss:

- Liability insurance
- Vicarious liability
- The anatomy of a lawsuit
- How to decrease your risk
- How to provide expert testimony

This chapter is meant only as an introduction to liability and in no way supercedes the need to consult with an attorney in the event of a clinician's actual involvement in a lawsuit.

LIABILITY INSURANCE

Liability insurance is purchased by clinicians and covers expenses incurred in the event the clinician is sued. Liability insurance may be viewed as a benefit for the employed clinician or as an expense for the clinician operating his or her own practice. Typically, the employed clinician negotiates liability insurance when discussing the employment contract. There are a few major points that a clinician should clearly understand when procuring liability insurance.

Who Pays the Premium?

Malpractice insurance premiums vary depending on the risk of the clinical specialty. Some areas of practice are much more likely to be associated with risk or generally have high awards for damages. Healthcare providers in higher-risk practices can expect to pay higher premiums for liability insurance. The premiums for nonphysician providers are generally lower than for physicians. Who is expected to pay these premiums should be clearly understood before the clinician's employment commences. Obviously, the clinician in private practice will pay his or her own premiums, but such clinicians also must consider who will pay the premiums of associates and employees.

Who Is Insured?

Liability policies generally cover a clinician in the course of his or her regular employment. The clinician may not be covered for an occurrence that happens in a department in which the clinician does not normally work. For instance, say that the clinician is visiting a friend who works in another department and offers to assist the friend with a procedure. If their actions result in an injury, the clinician may not be covered. Thus, the clinician must understand the policy's portability. Does the policy cover the clinician or the clinician's services? A company's liability insurance does not cover an employee who works at another practice, nor does it cover volunteer activities.

Is There a Deductible?

A deductible may apply to any case settled by the insurance company. The amount of the deductible should be ascertained up front and the clinician should know who is responsible for the deductible.

What Does the Insurance Cover?

Liability insurance generally covers a clinician practicing in his or her normal capacity. The policy may state that it covers the clinician in acts of negligence but not in acts of maliciousness. The clinician has a duty to report to his or her employer any incident that may result in a claim. Similarly, a clinician in private practice should notify his or her insurance company of any event that may precipitate legal action.

Under What Circumstances Do You Lose Coverage?

Policies may refuse coverage if the provider was impaired (under the influence of drugs or alcohol) when providing care. Liability insurance does not cover criminal activity, acting outside of one's scope of practice, tampering with records, or punitive damages. If a clinician is terminated from employment, who is responsible for purchasing tail coverage should be determined (see section on tail insurance).

What Are the Policy Limits?

Common coverage limits vary among specialties depending on the amount of risk generally assumed by the specialty area. The amount of the premium is directly proportional to the amount of coverage purchased. The policy will define the limits by (1) single occurrences and (2) multiple occurrences. For example, a policy that provides 1 million/3 million coverage provides up to 1 million dollars of coverage to the injured person and up to 3 million dollars of coverage to family members or others indirectly affected by the injury.

Tail Insurance

Tail insurance is purchased when a clinician leaves a practice or organization or switches insurance companies. Tail insurance covers occurrences that occurred during a clinician's tenure with the company and are filed after the clinician leaves the organization, switches insurance companies, or retires from clinical practice. Tail insurance may be purchased by the clinician, the organization he or she is leaving, or the new place of employment.

Supplemental Insurance

Practicing clinicians may want to consider purchasing supplemental insurance from the employers' insurance company if they work in high-risk fields in which awards generally are greater than the amount of the policy's limits.

VICARIOUS LIABILITY

Vicarious liability refers to the liability a collaborating physician assumes for the actions of a clinician. Depending on the licensure of the clinician, vicarious liability may be more of a myth than an actual threat. If the clinician is independently licensed and is granted authority to practice by state law under that license, the consulting physician is less likely to be held accountable for the clinician. Conversely, clinicians who practice under the licensure and authority of a physician are more likely to involve physicians in liability cases.

Physicians who employ clinicians may be more at risk for vicarious liability because employers are often held accountable for the actions of their employees. Even without an employee-employer relationship, a consulting physician who insists on co-signing each note or reviewing each chart containing documentation by the clinician is likely to be considered more accountable for the care provided by the clinician.

Physicians are also at risk for being held vicariously liable if they direct the clinician to perform tasks or procedures that are beyond the competency or scope of practice of the clinician.

Some physicians are reluctant to practice with nonphysician providers because they fear increasing their liability risk. This assumption is not statistically supported, however. A study by the American College of Obstetricians and Gynecologists noted that their physician members who practiced with nurse-midwives were *less likely* to be sued than their colleagues who did not work with midwives.[1]

Physicians who fear vicarious liability are often the same physicians who create barriers to the clinician's practice. If the physician insists that patients be admitted to a hospital under a physician, that prescriptions written by clinicians be filled in the physician's name, and that charts and notes be co-signed by a physician and the bill generated in the physician's name, is there any surprise that the clinician and physician are linked in liability?

THE ANATOMY OF A LAWSUIT

If a clinician employed by an organization or hospital is involved in a lawsuit, the institution will handle the process. The clinician is usually notified by the risk management department of the organization that an intent to serve notice has been received. Occasionally, the plaintiff (person initiating the lawsuit) may sue both the individual clinician and the organization, in which case the clinician may also receive a summons. If such a notification is received, the clinician must notify the risk management department immediately.

Clinicians in independent practice will be served a lawsuit via a summons. The clinician should notify his or her insurance company immediately when a summons is received. The clinician must present a copy of the summons to the insurance company and should receive a receipt from the insurance company that confirms that the insurance company received the summons.

Soon after the insurance company is notified of the summons, the clinician should receive a notification of coverage or denial of coverage from the insurance company. Whether covered by an institution's policy or an individual policy, the clinician *must cooperate with the insurance company in defending the lawsuit.*

The insurance company provides an attorney to defend the clinician. In some cases, the clinician may receive a letter notifying him or her that the estimated damages may exceed the policy limits. If this is the case, the clinician may wish to retain his or her own lawyer to monitor the situation.

The litigation process begins with a **period of discovery**. During this time, the lawyer will prepare for the defense of the clinician. The clinician must remain available for depositions and interrogatories. **Interrogatories** are written questions regarding the case that the clinician is required to answer. The clinician should also be available to assist the attorney with interpretation of the clinician's notes in the medical record. (A word of advice: The clinician can save him or herself a lot of grief by notifying his or her attorney of scheduled vacations and other obligations well in advance.)

In most states, both the plaintiff and defense attorneys must obtain **affidavits of merit**. These are attestations obtained from expert witnesses on each side that the case has merit. Unless a case has obvious conclusions (amputation of the wrong body part), a clinician can never be found liable in his or her field without another professional testifying against him or her. The testimonies of expert witnesses help to sort out the medical details of the case. Expert witnesses will be asked to comment on the **standard of care** that should occur in a particular situation. The standard of care is set by the time of the event in question. New technologies, medications, or therapies cannot be considered the standard of care for cases that predate their use. Because jurors are usually not medical professionals, they must depend on medical experts to provide information with which to decide a case.

In order for a case to proceed, four criteria must be met. The clinician must have a **duty** to provide services to the plaintiff, the plaintiff must prove there was a **breach of duty** on the part of the clinician, and **causation** (something the clinician did or failed to do) must be determined and result in **damage.**

The vast majority of malpractice cases are settled before the case goes to trial. A series of settlement attempts (states vary on the process) initially occur in efforts to resolve the case before a trial commences. The clinician should be warned that despite sound evidence that supports the position of the clinician, the cost of litigating a claim and the potential for loss may result in the two sides reaching a settlement prior to trial. Settlement is not necessarily an admission of guilt, but rather a mechanism to resolve the dispute. The insurance company generally has approval to settle a case without the consent of the clinician. In rare cases, when the deductible is high, a clinician may have approval rights with regards to settling a case.

Once the case is concluded, if damages are awarded, the occurrence is documented in the **National Data Bank** and is a matter of public record. Clinicians applying for subsequent positions of employment, clinical privileges, or malpractice insurance will be queried as to any previous litigation against the clinician. In cases where large awards are paid, the state may investigate the clinician and impose its own sanctions on the clinician's license independent of the lawsuit.

Involvement in a lawsuit is nerve-racking for even the most stalwart clinician. The clinician must rely on the advice of the insurance company and provide complete cooperation to bring a case to a close.

DECREASING YOUR RISK

Some healthcare providers believe that in today's society it is not a question of *if* one is sued, but *when*. Although there is no guarantee that one can avoid a lawsuit, there are a few simple rules a clinician can follow to decrease his or her risk.

Keep Practice Guidelines Up to Date

As discussed in previous chapters, the practice guidelines define the legal basis for a clinician's practice, describe the parameters or scope of practice, and describe situations in which the physician should be consulted. These guidelines should be updated regularly to reflect changes in practice and are part of a clinician's defense in the event of a lawsuit. Old guidelines must be kept because the guidelines in effect at the time of an occurrence are the ones the clinician is held to during examination of a case.

Practice Within the Scope of Practice

The clinician must practice within his or her scope of practice as defined by the practice guidelines. Deviation from the guidelines dramatically raises the risk for settlement in favor of the plaintiff. As discussed earlier, practice guidelines should not be so specific as to disallow individualized care or clinical judgment. Guidelines that are too stringent can also be damaging if the clinician opts for an alternative mechanism for care that is not included in the guidelines.

Consult a Physician Appropriately

When indicated, a physician must be consulted as the situation demands. Allegations against clinicians often include failure or a delay in obtaining physician consultation. The physician's response or instructions should be documented. Such consultation should be clearly documented in the medical record. The record should also reflect who is responsible for the management of the patient. If management of the patient is transferred from the clinician to the physician, the record should reflect the time of the transfer of responsibilities. A simple notation such as "Dr. X notified and assuming care of the patient" can serve to protect the clinician from liability resulting from further management.

Document Well

Because virtually all lawsuits occur well after the occurrence, the medical record is a vital piece of information that can support or condemn the clinician. Documentation should be clear, concise, accurate, and timely. Illegible documentation is a poor defense in a malpractice case. Informed consent and informed refusal are also important to document.

All documentation should be factual, but it is permissible, and often helpful, if the clinician documents his or her thought processes and differential diagnoses. Late entries are permissible, as long as the clinician indicates the time of the entry, but at no time is altering of the record allowed.

The recommendations presented in this section can decrease a clinician's risk of involvement in a lawsuit. In summary, the clinician should give the best, most consistent care he or she can in accordance with the scope of practice and provide sound documentation of the care given.

PROVIDING EXPERT TESTIMONY

At some point in the clinician's career, he or she may be asked to review a medical malpractice case and provide expert testimony. Clinician's are usually chosen for this role based on a personal or professional recommendation, previous experience with an attorney or law firm, or the clinician's reputation. Some states have enacted laws that require a clinician to have been in clinical practice at the time the occurrence took place.

The decision to perform in this capacity is entirely up to the individual clinician. If the clinician struggles with public speaking or is easily intimidated, this may not be the best avenue for expanding one's professional horizons. The potential expert witness must have an attention for detail, be considered an expert in his or her field, and have a flexible schedule.

Once the clinician agrees to serve in this capacity, he or she will be asked to submit to the attorney or law firm a curriculum vitae and a summary of fees the clinician will charge for his or her services. Fees usually include an hourly rate for review of materials and research, an hourly rate for depositions and testimony at trial, plus other expenses such as travel, phone calls, or missed work.

Providing expert testimony begins with a review of all relevant records regarding the case. The clinician should request a copy of the practice agreements because they represent an integral part of determining if the clinician involved in the lawsuit acted within his or her scope of practice. The attorney hiring the clinician may ask the clinician to sign a notarized affidavit of merit in order for the case to proceed. The clinician may be deposed in order to discuss his or her opinions concerning the case and may be sent depositions of other expert witnesses and those involved in the lawsuit as the case continues. The clinician will be instructed by the attorney on how to communicate or document his or her impressions of the case.

One of the most demanding aspects of serving as an expert witness is the provision of testimony at a trial. The clinician will be expected to travel to the site of the trial. Trials and testimonies are often cancelled, rescheduled, or delayed. Like the clinician involved in the lawsuit, the clinician serving as an expert witness should make the attorney aware of scheduled vacations and commitments well in advance.

The clinician is reminded that all information, records, depositions, and testimony are to be kept in the strictest confidence. When a case is resolved, the clinician must destroy all materials received involving the case in a manner that protects the privacy of all participants.

This chapter has addressed some of the key concepts surrounding medical malpractice. Although there is no guarantee that a clinician will be able to escape risk altogether, by employing a few key concepts the clinician may decrease his or her risk.

NOTE

1. ACOG Data, Survey of Professional Liability, American College of Obstetricians & Gynecologists, Washington DC. 1992, 1999.

CHAPTER 8

WORKING AND PLAYING WELL WITH OTHERS

It is never to the clinician's advantage to be adversarial in any form of practice. In Chapter 5 we discussed with whom it is important for the clinician to form professional relationships. These relationships help to establish an accurate understanding of who the clinician is and cultivate an environment in which the clinician can be a viable healthcare provider, community member, and professional. As stated in that chapter, people find it easier to be unreasonable and restrictive when the party in question is anonymous. They find it much more difficult to be close-minded concerning someone with whom they have shared a round of golf or a table at a cocktail party.

This chapter addresses those relationships within the healthcare team itself. No matter the definition or practice style of the healthcare provider, none of us stands alone as an island in the healthcare milieu. We all function interdependently with other professionals to achieve the most cost-effective, comprehensive, and safest care for those entrusting us with their care. Failure to function collaboratively with others in the healthcare arena does our patients a great disservice.

THE PHYSICIAN

At the top of the professional "food chain" is the physician. Some would argue this point, but I maintain that this is the entity with the most education, influence, responsibility, and control in the United States today with regards to health care. Society still embraces "the doctor" as the healthcare "god." In fact, consumers of health care that regularly receive services from clinicians who are not physicians still refer to their providers as "my doctor" and still attend "doctor's appointments."

Bearing this in mind, it would be unwise and downright foolish of the clinician to make an enemy of the physician. Would it not make better sense to work on the same side, taking advantage of the physician's position of influence? To do this, a relationship with a physician must be cultivated and nurtured. The clinician should not hide behind the physician, but instead become his or her partner and make use of the physician's influence. Among the most important advantages of a physician–clinician relationship is the opportunity to increase knowledge and skills.

In many cases, a relationship with at least one physician exists when the clinician begins practice. In some cases, such a relationship is required by law, in others it is an employer–employee relationship. In another scenario, the clinician and physician come together in a sort of "arranged marriage" through their mutual employment by the same organization. Whatever the basis or motivation for the relationship, the establishment of mutual trust and respect for one another is paramount to the success of the venture.

Trust, respect, honesty, communication—it does sound a bit like a marriage, doesn't it? In a marriage, both partners share responsibilities for the maintenance of the relationship. Each contributes uniquely, but in partnership, because mutual goals and aspirations are shared. Common interests are helpful in forming a relationship, but maintaining one's individuality also adds depth, value, and independence.

PHILOSOPHY

Once the clinician and physician can communicate in the same language regarding the skills and competency of the clinician, examination of each party's practice philosophy is important. Unshared or incongruent philosophies that clash rather than complement one another have the potential to create as much tension in a relationship as a marriage between two people of different religions. Often, differences in philosophy, such as high tech versus high touch, actually serve to strengthen a practice because each provider respects the unique contributions of the other and the practice can offer the best of both philosophies to its patients. Care is then delivered on a level that is appropriate to the needs of the patient.

THE COURTSHIP

When people establish a relationship, it is usually because of an initial attraction born out of common interests or circumstances. Courtship is a delicate dance that may start with surface enthusiasm, but as the relationship becomes more serious, a more in-depth evaluation of shared philosophies and beliefs occurs. The same is true for people contemplating a joint business venture or partnership. The clinician and physician must enter into discussions as to the nature of the relationship (the philosophy of care delivery) and arrive at a common understanding as to the role of each provider in the relationship. It will most likely be the burden of the clinician to educate the physician as to the value of the partnership. Because most physicians reflexively view the clinician as a competitor, the benefits of collaborating with the clinician should be discussed.

Revenue

The most obvious benefit of collaborating with a clinician is the increased revenue that the clinician can bring into the physician's practice. The cost of adding a nonphysician provider is less costly than adding another physician to a practice because salary and liability insurance are both considerably lower for a clinician. The clinician can manage routine care, thus allowing the physician to see more complex patients. The relief of the physician's workload also frees up more time for the physician to perform procedures and surgeries.

Another way to look at the financial gains of employing a clinician is the benefit of using the lower-cost clinician to generate the same revenue that a higher-priced physician once generated. When clinicians expand their skills, they add even more value to a practice. If the practice participates in contracts with insurance companies, managed care organizations, or state-funded programs that reimburse at rates less than gross charges, use of the less-expensive clinician helps to offset the cost of providing care to these individuals. This is not to say that all indigent patients should be assigned to clinicians who are not physicians. Sound ethical practice would assign patients to providers based on risk or acuity of the patient's complaint and the skills of the provider rather than the financial status of the patient. This enables the practice to see patients efficiently and cost effectively.

Referrals

Physicians who are willing to collaborate with clinicians automatically establish a source of referrals. Although the scope of practice varies from clinician to clinician, it is generally accepted that the services of a physician are required for those patients needing care that falls outside the expertise of the clinician. Clinicians with a large patient base provide the physician with a source for referrals.

Access

Another benefit of using clinicians is improved access to care. Patients often are dissatisfied with their inability to get appointments when they desire them. Offices that have a wait of 2 to 3 months for a routine appointment will begin to lose patients. When new patients are forced to wait several weeks for an appointment, they will often continue to shop for more accessible care. Overbooking that results in long wait times in the waiting areas or exam rooms also frustrates patients. The addition of more care providers increases a practice's ability to see more patients in a timely manner.

Satisfaction

Studies have shown that consumers who have received care from clinicians are extremely satisfied with the services. Appointments with nurse-practitioners, midwives, physicians assistants, and other such clinicians tend to be longer than appointments scheduled with physicians, and clinicians tend to deliver more personalized care.[1]

Quality

Physicians often view themselves as the protectors of the quality of health care. Some physicians believe it is their inherent responsibility to assure quality of care to all recipients. If they lack understanding of the education and scope of practice of the clinician, they may view the care of a clinician as inferior or they may deem it their responsibility to police or supervise the clinician to an unnecessary degree. Again, it becomes the duty of the clinician to educate the physician with respect to the competency of the clinician (see Chapter 11).

THE PRENUPTIAL AGREEMENT

Employment contracts were discussed in Chapter 6. For purposes of this discussion, we will discuss a document that is interchangeably referred to as the practice agreement or practice guidelines.

As discussed in Chapter 2, practice agreements differ from protocols. **Protocols** describe a process or procedure much in the same way a recipe book gives instructions for preparing a dish. **Practice guidelines** allow for individual assessment and management and the employment of clinical judgment. Protocols may exist within practice guidelines.

The practice guidelines may include a description of the legal basis for the practice, the scope of practice of the clinician, the responsibilities of the collaborating physician, and various appendices that may include protocols for procedures or drug formularies. Practice guidelines should be revised and updated regularly. Outdated copies should be archived because the practice guidelines also serve to delineate privileges and practice expectations in cases of liability. The practice guidelines in effect at the time care was given are those that are applicable in a liability case.

When clinical scenarios are addressed, practice guidelines are generally vague. This allows for individual assessment and the application of clinical judgment. If the guidelines are too stringent, the clinician is given very little flexibility in managing problems that may have a variety of treatment options. In this case, practice guidelines that do not allow for individualized care place the clinician and physician at increased risk for liability even if the care given is clinically sound or appropriate.

Many clinicians have their prescriptive authority delegated to them by a licensed physician. State laws often require that the clinician and the physician have a formal agreement as to the type and dosages of prescriptions that are delegated. Documentation of the collaborative agreements or formal relationship between the physician and the clinician also must exist. The practice guidelines are a logical place to provide such documentation.

In cases in which billing rights are assigned to a physician or practice and bills are generated in the physician's name (see "incident to" in Chapter 13), payors (insurance companies) may require the signature page of the practice guidelines be submitted as documentation that proves which clinicians are working with which physicians. The signature page is signed by each provider in the practice and is an attestation of the fact that the guidelines are a collaborative document developed and endorsed by those who have signed it.

Practice guidelines are a valuable tool when orienting new providers and should be available for newly hired professionals so that they can familiarize themselves with practice patterns and expectations. Professional students should also review the practice guidelines before beginning clinical work with a practice.

THE MARRIAGE

Once a relationship commences, it is the responsibility of all parties to commit to its maintenance. Of paramount importance is good communication. Disagreements and differences of opinion are common in any healthy relationship. Failure to communicate erodes the relationship and ultimately could create an unsafe environment for patients. As a relationship progresses, trust builds and providers can enjoy a satisfying professional relationship with all of the rewards discussed previously in this chapter.

When dissent does occur, discussions should take place privately; clinical providers must maintain an appearance of unity in front of staff members and patients. Failure to do so results in confusion and split loyalties and destroys the integrity of the providers.

THE WEDDING PARTY

Positive relationships between providers are essential to the well-being of any healthcare practice; however, relationships between the providers and support staff are equally important. Many people work very hard to contribute to the smooth operation of a practice (consider the number of staff required to keep a busy office running efficiently). Although a measure of respect is due providers given their inherent responsibility, staff members also deserve to be treated fairly and kindly.

When working with a clinician for the first time, the staff should be oriented to the role of the clinician. The clinician should meet with the staff and discuss briefly the legal basis for practice, the clinician's practice philosophy, and expectations regarding staff performance. When hiring staff, the clinician should keep in mind that staff who are cross-trained to perform multiple roles are very cost-effective, especially in a fledgling business.

The person answering the phone is perhaps the most important public relations person in the practice. This person should be pleasant, outgoing, and demonstrate a genuine affinity for people. This person should also exude confidence in the skills and qualifications of the clinician. The front-desk person also should be familiar with the office location and be able to provide clear directions to the practice.

If staff members are to perform at their best, the clinician should ensure that each person receives adequate training for the job that he or she is required to do. Staff members often are hired and trained in a "baptism by fire" that leaves everyone frustrated. Whenever possible, replacements should be hired before their predecessors leave so that proper orientation can take place before a staff member is expected to take full responsibility for filling a position.

Each provider performs procedures a little differently. Clinical assistants must be given time to assimilate all of the idiosyncrasies of each provider. A little patience and tolerance goes a long way in this situation to win the devotion of support staff. In very large offices, providers should attempt, whenever possible, to standardize procedures. Keeping track of large numbers of providers and their individual demands can stress staff members needlessly. Another solution would be to schedule support staff to work with one or two providers rather than rotate all of the staff through several providers.

Some offices provide a skeleton support staff to clinicians who are not physicians. These clinicians are expected to place their own patients in exam rooms, obtain and label their own specimens, take vital signs, and schedule appointments even though the physician employs several staff members for these functions. This situation limits the ability of the nonphysician provider to work at his or her full capacity because valuable billable time is spent performing these tasks. The clinician should have an open conversation with the physician or practice administrator to discuss productivity expectations and ways to improve process.

When considering hiring a new clinician, the office's current level of support staff should be evaluated. Failure to provide adequate support staff to a clinician thwarts the efforts of the practice to increase revenue or provide better access to care. When interviewing for a position, the clinician should ask about the amount of support that will be provided. If the clinician is expected to perform many support tasks that could be better handled by other staff members, productivity goals should be adjusted proportionately.

THE ENVIRONMENT

A comfortable and efficient work environment is essential to optimize clinical performance. If establishing one's own practice, the practitioner must examine local building codes as well as public health and fire codes. Zoning restrictions may also determine practice locations. The clinician also should consider conveniences such as proximity to facilities such as hospitals, laboratories, and radiology services. Be sure to allow for adequate parking and check for handicapped access.

Inside the office suite, the clinician should make sure that there is enough square footage to house all clerical and clinical operations. The clinician should ask the following questions:

- How many exam rooms per provider are available?
- Is there a need for a procedure room?
- How many offices are needed?
- Is there adequate storage?
- Will a laboratory be needed?
- Is a conference room necessary?
- Is the waiting area large enough to seat patients comfortably?
- How much office equipment will be needed?
- How many phone lines and computer terminals will be needed?
- Are there adequate restroom facilities?

These questions only begin to scratch the surface. The clinician should have a well-defined idea of what services will be provided and then consult other professionals to obtain advice about office floor plans. Providing care in less-than-adequate space with less-than-adequate equipment is quite challenging.

As a final examination, the clinician should view the office setting from the eyes and ears of the patient. Spend time sitting in the waiting room to learn what patients can hear or see from that vantage point. Spend a few moments in the examination room. Is the temperature warm enough for the patient in a paper gown? Does sound travel through the walls, compromising confidentiality?

The clinician hired into an organization or practice may be faced with some of the same questions. A minimum of two examination rooms per provider is necessary to keep the provider seeing patients. Otherwise, the clinician will spend time waiting for patients to dress and undress in a single examination room. Space for charting near the clinical area will prevent the provider from walking to and from an office to complete records. Examination rooms should be well stocked. Equipment or supplies needed for each visit should be anticipated and available in the examination room so that the clinician does not have to leave the room during a patient encounter or wait for an assistant to bring the necessary supplies.

When sterile procedures are performed, an assistant should be expected to remain in the room to assist with the procedure or obtain needed supplies. A chaperone is advised, especially when a clinician is examining or treating a member of the opposite sex. Some would argue a chaperone should be standard during all examinations.

In addition to clinical space, each clinician should have office space that is able to support the clerical work of the provider. Reference materials should be accessible. Phone lines and computer terminals may be needed, and privacy and quiet are a must if the clinician will be placing calls to patients from this area.

The well-functioning office is designed to meet the needs of the clinicians, their support staff, and the patients. Efforts to cut corners ultimately will result in decreased productivity, and therefore decreased revenue. Given the proper tools and environment, the practice can operate at maximum capacity to the satisfaction of the providers and their customers.

This chapter discussed the importance of building collegial work relationships to optimize patient care. Such relationships have many benefits both to providers and patients. "Arranged marriages" can work provided all parties are willing to take the time to explore one another's philosophies, tendencies, and prejudices and then work to build bridges constructed of respect, trust, and sometimes a little tolerance.

An environment that supports the physical needs of the practice and incorporates a well-trained support staff enables healthcare providers to deliver the highest quality of care to their patients.

NOTES

1. Choosing a Primary Care Provider, Health Central—General Encyclopedia, http://www.healthcentral.com/mhc/top/001939.cfm (accessed 1/2003).

Choosing a Primary Care Provider, Henry Ford Health Systems, http://www.henryfordhealth.org/12781.cfm (accessed 1/03).

Aiken, L. H., Achieving an Interdisciplinary Workforce in Healthcare, *New England Journal of Medicine,* 348(2003): 164–166.

CHAPTER 9

THE CAPITOL CONNECTION

The clinician who was intimidated by the chapter on rules and regulations (Chapter 2) cannot help but to develop a case of hives when faced with the challenge of political activism. However, if the public is generally ignorant of the scope of practice of the nonphysician provider, you should assume that the legislators representing the general public are just as uninformed. Yet, legislators make the laws we must live by. It is *vital* to the survival of the clinician's practice for the clinician to become and remain involved in politics from the local to the national level.

The clinician should begin by identifying his or her lawmakers. The township office, city hall, or county seat can provide a list of local, state, and federal legislators. Information can also be obtained at a post office, secretary of state's office, a local library, or government Web sites. The local or national organization representing the clinician will also maintain a list of legislators.

It is then important to schedule an appointment with the lawmaker to introduce yourself as a constituent and as a professional. Take along resource materials, including a fact sheet (one page) about your profession and a description of the people you serve. You may also want to include information produced by the national organization that represents your particular profession. Offer yourself as a local expert on issues that pertain to your practice. Make sure to take business cards to leave with the lawmaker and his or her staff. It is common to think that you will not get past the secretary at the door when attempting these visits, however, when appointments are scheduled in advance, legislators are more than willing to meet with constituents. Send a thank-you note and follow up with any information that the lawmaker requested during the visit.

Once you have made the acquaintance of your legislator, continue to contact him or her regularly (four to six times a year) to maintain the relationship. Consider volunteering during re-election time or host a social event or fundraiser in honor of the legislator. Once on the mailing list, you will be invited to events that will provide opportunities to interact with the legislator and other movers and shakers in the community. Watch for announcements about and invitations to community forums, town meetings, and other gatherings where you can see and be seen. These meetings are often attended by older males in the community. A new face is sure to attract attention. Establishing such relationships paves the way as you begin to develop or participate in a legislative agenda pertinent to your practice situation.

One of the perceived barriers that clinicians encounter is the threat of physician opposition to proposed legislation that allows for the expanded role of the clinician. Physician groups do have some advantages. They typically have money that supports lobbyists and large Political Action Committees (PACs) to protect their turf. Clinicians are perceived as a direct threat to traditional medicine. If clinicians gain acceptance as entry-level providers, the physicians' control of health care will be threatened. While physicians may honorably speak to the threat to quality of care and patient safety, it is often the threat to their income that is of primary concern.

Times are changing, and although it is not the intention of this book to bash physicians, some of their character traits work against them. The selfless physician of the past was seldom questioned or sued and was held in the utmost reverence by the general population. When medicine became more specialized, healthcare consumers and physicians alike embraced a more elitist attitude, which nearly led to the demise of the family doctor. People were willing to travel greater distances to see specialists. This change also brought about a disintegration of the physician–patient relationship. The physician no longer gave "cradle to grave" care for several generations of the same family, thus eroding the family–doctor relationship. Expectations changed; it was no longer necessary to be "nice," as long as one was "good." Similarly, for the physician, maintaining a professional distance allowed him or her to maintain his or her objectivity. This distancing from the patient has been viewed by many as arrogance.

As demands for healthcare reform have surfaced, physicians who have spent thousands of dollars and have given their lives to building lucrative practices are clinging tenaciously to the standard of healthcare delivery to which they have become accustomed. As more and more Americans find themselves among the uninsured or underinsured, a cry for change is being heard across the country. This, coupled with a declining economy and the emergence of managed care, has affected the physician's ability to produce revenue, causing physicians to feel even more threatened. In their attempts to protect their own interests, physicians are often viewed by legislators as self-serving, whereas nonphysician providers are seen as more trustworthy and as having the well-being of their patients as their primary concern. The clinician's reputation for caring for those patients "who no one else wants" is serving the profession well.

Take heart though, a new breed of physician is emerging. Collaboration without control will be the model of the future. More physicians are practicing in large, multispecialty groups that allow the physician to enjoy a more predictable lifestyle. More women are entering health care because it is now possible to blend motherhood and medicine. The practice of medicine is no longer above scrutiny or shrouded in mystique as it has been in the past. Health care has become more competitive as consumers are shopping for care that is satisfying as well as competent.

Bearing in mind these changes in public opinion with regards to medical care and the traditionally egocentric focus of the American Medical Association, the legislative agenda of the clinician should focus on issues such as access to care, health maintenance, quality, and reduced cost. Lawmakers will most likely turn a deaf ear to clinicians clamoring for political justice.

Legislative agendas cost time and money. It behooves the clinician to become aligned with an organizing body that represents others with similar interests. Most clinicians are represented by a national organizing body that, in turn, has local or regional chapters. These local chapters have a responsibility to stay politically abreast of issues affecting the clinician's profession with help from the national office as needed. Developing relationships with organizations that share common interests can result in the pooling of resources and shared agendas.

Consumer groups that may support the clinician's practice can be of valuable help when promoting legislation. Members of these groups are available to write letters, stuff envelopes, testify, or otherwise aid in the cause of the clinician. It is an even greater advantage if the members of this group are voting constituents of the targeted lawmakers. Incidentally, nonphysician providers may feel that their numbers are too small to generate legislators' interest; however, the large numbers of patients cared for by these clinicians represent an impressive body of voters.

Once a legislative initiative has been identified, the group supporting a bill or proposed change must prepare to introduce the bill. The following steps can help you organize your campaign.

- Prepare a fact sheet. This is a one-page statement about who you are and what you do. Be complete, but concise.
- Prepare a position statement. Define one problem per statement and explain how it affects public health. Describe your position and how you can help.
- Prepare testimony. Testimony is usually prepared using an introduction or statement of the problem and "talking points" or points you wish to make during your testimony.
- Contact lawmakers. Legislators who may be willing to introduce or support your bill should be contacted and made familiar with your position.

Logically, legislators who serve on committees relevant to your bill would be a priority to contact. For example, legislators on the health policy committee in your state would be a good starting point for most legislation affecting health care and clinicians.

Once a sponsor has agreed to introduce your bill, you will need to contact others who may be willing to support the bill. After a bill is introduced, it will be assigned to a committee that, after investigation and perhaps testimony, will make a recommendation on passing or defeating the bill. Once approved by the committee, the bill goes to the house or senate floor (depending on where it was introduced) for a vote. (Some bills go through the policy process in both chambers concurrently.) Once approved by both chambers, the bill goes on to the governor to be signed into law.

Many entities employ a lobbyist to assist with the legislative process. A lobbyist, albeit an expensive investment, works diligently through the legislative process on behalf of those contracting his or her services. Most clinicians cite a busy schedule as the primary reason they are not politically active. When family and other outside activities are compounded with the demands of a clinical schedule, there is little time to run off to the state capitol to lobby politicians.

A lobbyist works on behalf of a group to support their political agenda. Your lobbyist helps you prepare your testimony, attends hearings with you, and conveys your message to legislators. The lobbyist continuously assesses the political climate and attains and maintains key contacts and relationships with lawmakers. The lobbyist keeps abreast of activity in the government and notifies you when political action on behalf of the members in your group is necessary. A lobbyist does not do all of the work, but the lobbyist is able to keep his or her finger on the pulse of the legislature and let you know when action is appropriate.

A lobbyist never takes the place of a clinician when your presence is required, however. It is *you* that the legislators want and need to hear from. If you are not committed enough to support your own agenda, it is unlikely that you will find legislative support. For those clinicians who are unwilling or unable to devote time to a legislative initiative, support those of your profession who are willing or able to commit time to politics. Donate money to your organization's Political Action Committee (PAC) and pay your dues to a professional membership that represents your clinical specialty. Donate to your legislator's campaign and take a few moments to write a card or letter to let that legislator know about your position on a particular issue.

Many clinicians complain bitterly about prejudice, barriers to practice, and public ignorance, yet are unwilling to do something about it. The laws will not change themselves. It takes the work of committed individuals who take the time to make a difference. Because all stand to gain from advances in legislation, all members of a group should play a role in carrying forth a political agenda.

The clinician in the twenty-first century is in a position to change health care in the United States. With their inherent philosophy about health maintenance and disease prevention and hands-on approach to healthcare delivery, clinicians can provide comprehensive, satisfying care within a model that delivers quality care efficiently and cost-effectively. But in order for that to happen, legislative changes must occur that will remove the barriers to practice that many clinicians face today.

CHAPTER 10

WHO AM I?

The focus of this book has been on business concepts for the clinician. It was written based on the premise that although clinicians are well educated in the clinical areas in which they practice, they often are not prepared adequately to enter the world of business. Many concepts in this book presumably would be of interest to physicians because they also receive very little education in basic business during medical school and their residency. Assuming that all healthcare providers begin at the same level of understanding (or ignorance) of business concepts, why then do nonphysician providers seem to have to work harder to reach the same goals that physicians appear to attain more easily?

One of the most obvious differences is the fact that there are few misunderstandings of the role, education, or authority of physicians. In fact, many times the body of knowledge of a particular physician is presumed by the general public to be much greater than it actually is. The general public does not contemplate the cardiologist's inability to perform neurosurgery or the obstetrician's unfamiliarity with chemotherapeutic agents. State licensure does not limit a physician's scope of practice to one specialty or another.

Conversely, public awareness and understanding of the role of the nonphysician ranges from a sense of uncertainty regarding the competency of such clinicians to the assumption that they are mini-doctors with similar skills. At any rate, the term *nonphysician* says a lot. Because the labels applied to these clinicians were discussed in an earlier chapter, we will not belabor these points now. Instead, the challenge is to the clinician: Who am I?

ADOPT A DEFINITION

Defining and articulating clearly the professional role and scope of practice of the clinician will at times become necessary to the clinician's survival. It will also be a prerequisite for any planned marketing or public relations efforts. Otherwise, the clinician should prepare to be forever misunderstood, or even worse, undervalued. State and national organizations representing the clinician may have published definitions that the clinician can use to describe his or her profession and practice.

ADOPT AN IDENTITY

The definition of the clinician helps to define his or her professional identity. If clinicians continue to remain nameless, they will remain invisible. The only way to combat ignorance is through education. When the clinician interacts with other members of the healthcare team, he or she begins to establish a professional identity by gaining the respect of other healthcare colleagues. These interactions serve to introduce the clinician as a competent, educated professional. Further interactions solidify the clinician as a member of the healthcare team.

KNOW THE RULES

Once the clinician can define his or her identity, the clinician can begin to develop a practice based on the legal basis for practice. The clinician must obtain the required credentials to practice in a state according to the rules and regulations in that state (see Chapter 2). Substantial knowledge regarding the rules and regulations as they pertain to the clinician is the clinician's responsibility. The clinician should research rules and regulations independently and not rely solely on others' interpretation of the law.

State laws also differ with respect to different categories of clinicians. It is common for administrators or physicians to confuse one type of nonphysician with another or to lump all clinicians who are not physicians into one category, assuming that the rules for one apply to all. The clinician should be prepared to cite state law as it pertains to his or her practice, clinical specialty, and licensure.

DEFINE YOUR PATIENT POPULATION

Clinicians commonly have a clinical focus or specialty area of practice just as physicians do. As the clinician attempts to clarify his or her role, he or she should prepare to answer the following questions: What is the target patient population(s)? Is care provided to only women, only men, only children, only couples who are infertile? Does the clinician specialize in adolescent care, substance abuse, or mental health? Clinicians who are not physicians can be found in virtually all areas of health care, and just as physicians differ in their education and clinical focus, so does the clinician.

DEFINE THE SCOPE OF PRACTICE

Once the clinician's identity, patient population, legal regulations, and clinical focus have been determined, the clinician can describe his or her scope of practice. To assist with this, the clinician can describe areas of practice where he or she has special skills or expertise. The clinician should describe any special interests or experience in a particular disorder or treatment and identify any practice philosophies that are unique. Defining these differences may give a clinician the competitive edge when it comes to marketing his or her practice.

ACT LIKE A PROFESSIONAL

Although a collaborative relationship with a physician is very desirable, and some clinicians are dependent on physicians for licensure, the clinician should take care to establish an identity separate from the physician's. This not only helps the clinician to establish his or her credibility as a healthcare provider, but also avoids confusion in some instances of patient care.

For example, suppose that a clinician wishes to consult a cardiologist after detecting a heart murmur during a routine physical exam of a patient. An impatient clerk in the cardiologist's office insists that she be given the name of the *physician* referring the patient to her employer. After the cardiologist evaluates the patient, she sends a letter to the *physician* with an impression and advice for further care. Even though it may be necessary, for billing purposes, to supply a physician's name in obtaining a consultation (some insurance companies do not recognize or credential a nonphysician provider), the clinician can establish him or herself as the care provider by dictating a letter to the cardiologist introducing the patient and formally requesting the consult. The cardiologist will then begin to view the clinician as a professional separate from the clinician's physician. The cardiologist will then gain an appreciation for the clinical skills and capabilities of the clinician.

The clinician should always take the time when referring to or consulting with a physician to personally call the physician to discuss the case or write a letter requesting the consult. This is not only good communication, but it offers the opportunity to collaborate with another healthcare provider. Many clinicians have won the respect of reticent physicians by collaborating appropriately and professionally.

WORK WITH THE SYSTEM

Laboratory and radiology reports ordered by a clinician that must be requested in a physician's name frustrate providers and patients alike. Results go to the physician who has never seen the patient instead of to the clinician ordering the tests. Many times these regulations result from insurance rules that require procedures or tests be ordered in a physician's name in order to bill and receive reimbursement for the services. Although this is a legitimate problem, the clinician should examine ways to include both the physician and the nonphysician provider on these forms.

Prescriptions written by a clinician but filled in the name of a physician confuse patients. The patient may be uncertain whether they have the right medication if he or she does not recognize the physician's name. To avoid confusion, the clinician can alert the patient that prescriptions may be labeled with the physician's name.

Pharmacists should be made aware of a clinician's practice in the community and about the clinician's legal prescriptive rights. A letter of introduction to local pharmacies with a business card attached serves to introduce the clinician to the pharmaceutical community.

BE A TEAM PLAYER

The clinician should also be able to articulate his or her role and scope of practice as it relates to other members of the healthcare team. Nurses in a labor and delivery unit may be confused about their role when midwives join an organization. Office staff members may feel confused and see the clinician as another layer within the office hierarchy. The clinician should be able to describe to other members of the healthcare team how he or she fits into the structure of an office or other clinical setting.

BE INDISPENSABLE

It is very important for clinicians to have a mechanism to determine what value they contribute to an organization, bearing in mind that value is not always measured in dollars and cents. Does the clinician participate in community education offerings sponsored by the organization? Does the clinician perform rape counseling? Is there a need that the clinician can fill that has previously been unmet? Does the clinician perform sports physicals for the local schools or volunteer at a free clinic? Is the clinician educating nursing students, medical students, or other fledgling professionals? Is the clinician available after hours to triage phone calls and prevent unnecessary visits to the emergency room? Is the clinician's patient satisfaction measured and found to be higher than that of other providers or meet institutional benchmarks or practice goals?

The clinician can also demonstrate fiscal responsibility within the practice by contributing to cost containment by using fewer resources when care is provided. Does the clinician's practice result in lower costs and better outcomes? The clinician should be cognizant of the value he or she brings to a practice and keep the data handy to share when appropriate.

BE PREPARED

The clinician must develop templates that answer these questions concisely and comprehensively. Whether it is a threat to practice or a marketing opportunity, the clinician must be able to rapidly assess a situation and determine what information to share, how much to share, and how to present it (see Chapter 12).

The clinician should always carry business cards and make them available so that he or she can be contacted for further information or located by a potential customer. The clinician should maintain a file of pertinent documents or articles that support his or her profession or position. The national or local organizing body can help supply the clinician with the documents necessary for conducting good business.

WHO AM I?

Because the clinician is commonly mislabeled, misunderstood, or pigeonholed in a single category with clinicians of other specialties, it is his or her responsibility to be able to clearly articulate who they are and what they do. The clinician should be the resident expert on his or her profession. Dependence on an employer or administrator to defend or describe the clinician and his or her scope of practice will often result in frustration and misinformation. It is often unrealistic to expect the organization's attorney to know about all the state rules and regulations pertaining to practice.

In summary, all clinicians are not educated or licensed equally. Confusion about the variety and differing roles and practice patterns of clinicians exists among physicians, administrators, legislators, and most important, customers. So, clinician, whenever someone strikes up a band, be prepared to toot your own horn!

CHAPTER 11

THE MARK OF EXCELLENCE

Health care is considered to be a service-oriented industry. For those professionals choosing to make a career of teaching, healing, and shepherding their patients through life's natural processes and infirmities, the rewards are many. Despite the satisfaction most healthcare providers feel in their chosen profession, most will admit to coping with a moderate to high level of stress due in part to the small margin of error allowed in the performance of their jobs. Although human error is accepted as inevitable, in the healthcare arena expectations are high and tolerance for error is extremely low.

The clinician, by virtue of being a *non*physician, can expect a fair amount of scrutiny when it comes to practice. Because the provision of health care for many years has been the domain of the physician, confidence in any other type of healthcare provider may be cautiously withheld. The clinician must remember that actions often speak much louder than words. If public opinion is to be changed, it will require the clinician to set an irrefutable track record for providing clinical care of the highest quality. By demonstrating excellence in practice, the clinician will earn the respect and endorsement of patients, peers, and physicians.

This chapter will discuss mechanisms for demonstrating and evaluating clinical competency. This is a four-step process that includes:

1. Defining the scope of practice
2. Defining the standard of care
3. Identifying clinical benchmarks
4. Participating in quality management and process improvement

DEFINING THE SCOPE OF PRACTICE

No professional performs his or her job in exactly the same way. The same holds true for healthcare professionals. In this book, the term **scope of practice** is used many times. This term refers to the limits or lines of demarcation that define what a given clinician can do. These lines are not hard and fast walls, but rather an undulating border that is shaped and reshaped during the course of the clinician's career.

If one imagines the ripples created when a stone is tossed into a pool, one could theorize that scope of practice resembles such an image. The student has a narrow scope of practice that widens with experience, and each ring of the circle indicates a new level of expertise gained as time passes and longevity increases. This rather simplistic description, though logical, is not accurate.

Just as scope of practice differs from one healthcare professional to the next, healthcare providers within the same specialty define their scope of practice differently. Professional organizations that represent clinicians purposefully are vague when describing scope of practice because it is recognized that no clear definition exists that applies to all clinicians, even those within the same area of clinical practice. But no matter the clinical focus, the clinician's scope of practice is redefined continuously by many variables. These variables may be either extrinsic or intrinsic, but it is the combination that adds up to complete the total picture.

The physician relationship has a strong influence on scope of practice. Because the physician often serves as a colleague and mentor, he or she has the ability to influence the development of the clinician's clinical skills and expertise. If the physician is progressive and innovative, the professional colleague is likely to be so as well. If the physician is a subspecialist, such as a reproductive endocrinologist, the women's health nurse-practitioner working with him or her will possess skills that other nurse-practitioners of similar training will not.

Physician practices that work with other clinicians and value their contributions to health care tend to be supportive and collaborative, often advocating on behalf of the clinician when necessary. Although the clinician may not always be able to select the consulting physician, whenever a match in skill and philosophy is found, all involved benefit.

The environment in which a clinician works also strongly defines scope of practice. If a clinician works in a rural setting, miles from the nearest physician or medical center, his or her scope of practice may differ from the clinician who works in a university teaching hospital. The resources available within such institutions affect how the clinician delivers care. Nurse-anesthetists, for example, practice under the direct supervision of anesthesiologists in regional care centers, yet may be the only provider delivering anesthesia in a small community hospital. A family nurse-practitioner may see essentially well patients and treat acute minor illnesses in an office setting or perform rounds and facilitate admissions in the inpatient setting. Thus, the setting in which a professional delivers care plays a role in defining the scope of practice.

It is well recognized that experience is a great teacher. Perhaps one of the greatest influences on scope of practice is the past experiences of the clinician. Although longevity definitely plays a major part in shaping the practice of a clinician, experience extends beyond the expertise and proficiency gained by longevity. Clinicians are unable to experience all scenarios within the same time frame, and some clinical situations are indeed rare. Therefore, each clinician will progress through his or her clinical career in a slightly different way than others who share his or her profession. Similarly, because outcomes are not predictable, clinicians will base their interpretations of similar clinical situations on different endings to similar stories.

Personal philosophy as well as religious and cultural beliefs will also serve to shape a clinician's habits and preferences, as will the inherent personality of the clinician. The clinician who is more of a risk taker will act and react differently in clinical situations than the clinician with a more conservative personality. Many clinicians rely on intuition in clinical practice, whereas others base each decision and action on a multitude of carefully evaluated facts. The well-rounded clinician employs a combination of fact and intuition when delivering care.

A clinician's scope of practice may vary from practice setting to practice setting depending on the variables discussed thus far. A clinician with prior experience in an organization may be denied privileges in another organization due to the lack of resources of the second organization or differences in bylaws or practice agreements. In situations like these, the clinician is advised to follow policies and protocols to the letter. If the clinician is frustrated by limitations these policies place on his or her practice, the clinician should work to revise the policies. The clinician should work to affect change within the system, but he of she should never circumvent it.

In summary, the scope of practice of each clinician cannot be categorized and defined in the strictest of terms, but instead is defined by the prevailing winds of a multitude of variables and the ways in which the clinician adjusts the sail.

DEFINING STANDARD OF CARE

If scope of practice is so poorly defined, how is it possible then to determine clinical excellence or standard of care? The **standard of care** is often incorrectly assumed to be the *ideal* way to provide care. Instead, standard of care is defined through evidence-based practice and clinical experience. Some standards are defined by groups such as the American Academy of Pediatrics. Such a group would define, for example, the immunization schedule for newborns. The clinician should consult local and national organizations to become familiar with standards set forth by such groups.

In other cases, the standard of care refers to what is geographically acceptable or what a reasonable clinician of similar training and background would do in a similar situation in a similar practice setting. Thus, standard of care, like scope of practice, is often difficult to define. The clinician would be wise when entering a new practice to become familiar with the local standard of care as it applies to his or her practice.

In cases of medical malpractice, the provider must demonstrate that he or she performed his or her duties according to the accepted standard of care. One of the roles of the expert witness in a malpractice case is to evaluate whether the provider met the standard of care. Because the standard of care may differ slightly between different types of healthcare providers, expert witnesses are generally asked to speak to the standard of care of those professionals they are qualified to evaluate. For example, a clinician could not speak to the standard of care of a physician.

IDENTIFYING CLINICAL BENCHMARKS

As just discussed, the standard of care defines common practice. **Benchmarking,** a new buzzword in clinical practice, is the process of identifying *best practices.* **Benchmarks** are statistical measures that are used in benchmarking. Benchmarking[1] began in Japan. In the United States, Xerox led the way in benchmarking in industry in 1979. The process of benchmarking was embraced by the healthcare field in the 1980s.

Benchmarking can be used as a part of the quality improvement process whereby a process or outcome considered to be of value is chosen to be benchmarked. A method of measuring the outcome is developed, the process is evaluated, and the best practices are identified. After identifying the best practices, the processes are explored to determine what interventions have been implemented to achieve the desired outcome.

For example, the standard of care recommends that all female patients be offered a screening mammogram by age 40. All of the primary care practices in an organization are evaluated for compliance with this standard. A chart audit identifies that the range of compliance is 30% to 85%. The practice with 85% compliance is identified, and its processes are evaluated to determine if other practices can employ its techniques to achieve higher rates of compliance. The clinician should be aware that certain variables may affect benchmarks, for instance, in our example, imagine if one of the primary care offices is able to provide mammography in their office. This situation may not be replicable in all of the other offices. Thus, in benchmarking, the highest score may not be a realistic goal for all practices. Conversely, if the office with the best rate of screening mammograms sends reminder cards to all patients due for an annual checkup, provides education about the value of mammography during the visit, and schedules the procedure for the patient at the end of the visit, this process could be implemented by other practices to improve results.

When a practice participates in benchmarking, its processes are continuously evaluated. Benchmarking also heightens awareness of a practice's actual performance as compared to other practices and can motivate a practice to initiate and implement change. Benchmarking results in a higher quality of care delivery.

The clinician should be familiar with the clinical benchmarks that are unique to his or her area of practice. By evaluating his or her practice against other practices, the clinician can validate that the care given is of the best quality or become aware that change is needed.

QUALITY MANAGEMENT AND PROCESS IMPROVEMENT

Most clinicians have heard of quality management or process improvement. Organizations have even used mnemonics such as PDCA (plan, do, check, act) to remind employees how to employ process improvement. If the clinician is a part of a large organization, committees may be formed for the express purpose of monitoring quality. With quality management and process improvement, specific quality indicators are identified. When clinical situations are identified according to the indicators, the management process is evaluated to determine if the care of the patient was appropriate. Often the committee may seek the input of the healthcare provider when the thought process or details of the case are not apparent from a chart review.

The purpose of quality management is primarily educational, not punitive. Cases are often tracked to determine if a pattern exists for a certain provider or process, but the primary concern of quality management is to learn from the experience and evaluate the current processes to determine if change is indicated.

All clinicians should be a part of the quality management process. Participation in quality management is often a requirement for hospital privileges. Because physicians are not always familiar with the practice patterns of other providers, it is useful to have clinical expertise from all areas of practice participating in quality management.

In the outpatient or ambulatory care setting, practices should employ an internal mechanism for quality management and process improvement. Indicators pertinent to the practice specialty or demographics of the patient population can be identified and evaluated quarterly or may be significant enough to require regular review. At any rate, a process that focuses on improving or maintaining quality of care should be the goal of all clinical settings.

By implementing some form of benchmarking, evaluation of process is not limited to the scrutiny of adverse outcomes, but also proactively strives to achieve and maintain clinical excellence in a practice.

In summary, the role or scope of practice of the clinician may vary widely from other clinicians and is dependent on a multitude of variables. The clinician should practice within the standard of care for his or her clinical specialty, which may differ slightly from one practice setting to another. The goal of any clinician should be to deliver the highest quality of care. Participating in benchmarking, quality management, and process improvement will assist the clinician in achieving this goal.

NOTE

1. Benchmarking: An overview—The Theme for the Nineties, http://www.agility.com.au/benchmark-frame.htm (accessed 3/2003).

CHAPTER 12

PLAYING THE NUMBERS

In Chapter 11, benchmarking and quality assurance were discussed as measures of quality of care and process improvement. There is no argument that the clinician should always strive for clinical excellence. In order to participate in activities such as quality improvement and benchmarking, the clinician must create a data set that provides the statistics necessary to evaluate clinical activity.

We have already established that most clinicians are not necessarily comfortable being politicians, it also is safe to assume that most clinicians do not consider themselves statisticians either. The demands of clinical work and full schedules do not allow much time for data gathering.

However, the clinician must create and maintain several data sets that support and protect his or her practice. Consider the hardworking clinician who is approached by the physicians in the practice and informed that she is being let go because she is not making money for the practice or the clinician who is considering hiring a partner but needs to know if the practice can support another provider.

"Playing the numbers" needs to be on every clinician's professional agenda. As mentioned in the discussion on benchmarking, data exist that can be used to measure outcomes and other clinical parameters, patient satisfaction, and financial performance. Taking a head-in-the-sand approach can be very costly to the clinician who remains ignorant of the data generated by his or her practice. The clinician must also develop a sense of what data are collected and with whom and when it is shared.

COST MEASURES AND PRODUCTIVITY

Employers, whether they are physicians, organizations, or the clinicians themselves, will be interested in several data sets generated by the work of the clinician. At the top of this list will of course be productivity. A more detailed discussion on the various ways to measure productivity is presented in Chapter 14. At any rate, an employer wants to know that each person in a practice is doing his or her job, and in the case of clinicians, generating revenue to sustain the practice.

Beware to the clinician who cannot state with a fair degree of accuracy how much revenue he or she generates in a month, a quarter, or a year. The clinician who is ignorant of this information is at risk of being undervalued, which is often manifested by decreased compensation or loss of a job. The clinician who generates three times his or her salary in billed revenue is generally considered productive. This figure may be a bit aggressive for a brand new clinician. If a clinician does not carry a full clinical load, but spends time in an administrative or faculty role, the proportion of salary to billed revenue will also be different.

Retrieving information on billed revenue may be more difficult for some clinicians than others. Some of the difficulties are created by the fact that bills for nonphysician providers are often submitted in the physician's name. If such is the case, an internal mechanism for delineating which charges result from the work of a physician versus the work of a nonphysician colleague should be developed.

Once the problem of separating charges by healthcare provider is solved, simply adding patient encounters by CPT codes and applying the charges for each code yields the **gross revenue** charged by each clinician. The clinician may at first be surprised by the amount of revenue that he or she is able to produce. The clinician must remember that this number represents gross charges. From that number, the clinician must subtract the costs of providing the service (or practice expenses) such as office rent, medical supplies, utilities, support staff salaries and benefits, and the providers' salaries, benefits, and liability insurance. Subtracting practice expenses from the gross revenue represents the **net revenue** generated by the practice.

CONTRACTING HEALTHCARE

Contractual allowances affect the amount of net revenue generated. **Contractual allowances** are agreements that have been made to provide a service for contract members for a set amount that may be less than what is normally charged for a service. The clinician may wonder why anyone would enter into such an agreement. The reason is that in today's competitive environment, healthcare providers may compete for contracts, especially from businesses that employ large groups of people. Contracting a large volume at a reduced rate rather than a smaller volume at a higher rate is good business.

It may be the mission of an organization to provide care to the indigent or to participate in plans that pay poorly, thus ensuring care for vulnerable populations. These contracts may result in a collection rate of less than half what is billed. It is not necessarily bad business to provide care at such a loss, providing that such arrangements are fulfilling the organization's mission to provide indigent care. The practice must also consider the bad debt write-off and subtract that from the billed revenue.

Each year, when it is time to reconsider contracts with payors, a practice must evaluate whether it wishes to continue to participate in the agreement. The contract should be carefully scrutinized to assure that no changes have been written into it that will adversely affect the practice. If the practice declines to continue participating with the payor, they **de-par,** or **departicipate,** from the plan. Patients covered by the plan have the choice of selecting another care provider who does accept, or **par,** with their insurance or continuing care with the practice and paying out of pocket for the services.

One of the considerations that a practice must evaluate is the number of patients that are covered by the plan. Departicipating from a plan that covers 30% of the practice's patients may not be wise. Instead, the practice may search for ways to deliver care more cost effectively, like . . . hiring a clinician for instance! Consider the original formula that subtracts practice expenses from revenue; if the provider's salaries and benefits, including liability insurance, are less, then this move would have a favorable impact on a practice's budget.

QUALITY MEASURES

A nonphysician provider, no matter how productive, would be a practice liability if the quality of care delivered was not maintained. Thus, in addition to productivity, the clinician should consider measures that evaluate quality of care. These clinical measures will differ from clinician to clinician, depending on the area of health care in which the clinician practices, but in most cases, each clinical specialty will recognize certain clinical parameters that are considered standard of care for that particular area of heath care. National benchmarks for health care also exist is certain clinical areas (see Chapter 11).

Clinical competence is not generally rewarded because it is considered mandatory; however, incompetence has its negative rewards, and the clinician should take care to document safe clinical practice. Some outcomes can favorably reflect on the clinical practice of providers. For example, low cesarean section rates, birth weights within normal ranges, and few neonatal intensive care admissions would reflect well on midwifery care. Positive outcomes such as these have both clinical and economic benefits.

The cost of delivering care is often as much of a concern to an insurance company as it is to a clinical practice. If an obstetrics practice boasts of a low cesarean section rate, this translates into the provision of obstetric care at less cost to the plan's members. This results from the fact that vaginal deliveries use fewer hospital resources and require shorter hospital stays. The medical leave of absence for the mother is shorter, thus decreasing time away from work. Complications from vaginal deliveries are less frequent and less serious than those that may arise from cesarean delivery, further decreasing costs.

Each area of clinical practice can apply their own scenarios that show where the health maintenance activity of the practice has had an impact on the cost of care delivery as well as clinical outcomes. Such data becomes valuable when negotiating contracts with a managed care organization or other insurance company. Many large companies are self-insured and will seek contracts with health systems that have proven themselves cost-effective, as well as clinically excellent.

Obtaining data that quantify quality of care and cost-effectiveness may be more difficult for some than others. Large organizations often employ outcomes coordinators that gather and evaluate data for just this reason. In smaller, independent practices, such data may result from individual chart reviews. Computer databases have been created for this purpose as well. Each clinician should do his or her share in collecting data, because each clinician stands to benefit from the rewards of documenting quality, cost-effective health care.

PATIENT SATISFACTION

Another data set of increasing importance when evaluating the delivery of healthcare are those that measure patient satisfaction. Again, as health care has become competitive and *patients* have become *consumers,* more attention has been given to measuring patient satisfaction. Among the points typically evaluated in terms of patient satisfaction are waiting time, accessibility of appointments, phone calls, perceived competence of providers, privacy issues, and respect shown to the patient.

Several methods for evaluating patient satisfaction are employed, including phone interviews by a contracted agency, exit surveys, mail surveys, and other tools. Whatever the method, each practice should measure patient satisfaction and use the resulting data in some form of process improvement that will increase patient satisfaction. No practice can afford the bad press generated by dissatisfied patients. A high level of patient satisfaction is attractive to managed care organizations and other consumers of health care.

DATA COLLECTION

Once the practice or organization has defined what data will be gathered, methods for data collection and the maintenance and dissemination of data will need to be determined. There may also be data in addition to that collected by an organization or practice that individual clinicians may feel is of value. Data should not be collected and then never evaluated. Data collection is labor intensive and of no value to anyone if the results are not reviewed regularly, but what is shared, when, and with whom needs to be considered.

SHARING DATA

The board of trustees of a hospital may be somewhat bored with episiotomy rates in a midwifery service but be on the edge of their seats when discussing practice growth and the bottom line. The local childbirth educators will not care one bit about a practice's financial solvency but salivate over a 10% episiotomy rate. As illustrated here, when sharing statistics, it is important to know the audience and their focus of interest.

A private hospital may not be particularly concerned about cesarean section rates because increased length of stay and use of the operating suite ultimately translates into more revenue. However, a hospital serving a largely indigent population whose state health insurance program reimburses the hospital the same for a cesarean as for a vaginal birth will be very interested in hearing about low cesarean section rates. The same holds true for a large employer evaluating competing health plans. Practices that have a reputation for health maintenance activity that decreases hospital admissions, such as outpatient diabetes care or free blood pressure screening visits, will be attractive to an employer, even more so if this is coupled with reports of good patient satisfaction. However, this employer will not be interested in the practice's demonstrated fiscal growth over the last quarter.

EMPLOYMENT CONTRACTS

Securing managed care contracts and impressing the hospital board of trustees should be important to clinicians, but the data that reflect personally on the individual clinician also are important. When negotiating a contract, the clinician is empowered if he or she is backed up by data that demonstrate a combination of clinical excellence, cost-effectiveness or cost containment, and patient satisfaction.

Sadly, many clinicians do not have access to data that they could use to interpret their value to a practice or organization. Sometimes this is out of ignorance as to the value of such data, but other times it is due to the employer or senior members of the practice withholding such information. This may be due to the fact that the practice owners may feel that the clinician has no right to such data and treats the clinician like other employees in the practice. As stated in Chapter 6, an agreement regarding profit sharing or partnership should be reached when a clinician joins a practice. Another reason for practice owners not to share productivity data with the clinician could be that the clinician is generating several times his or her income and the practice administrators prefer the clinician not know this!

Some organizations depend on regional trends to determine salaries. The difficulty with this method, as mentioned previously, is that all providers are not practicing in the same way. The nonphysician provider may have to perform research to determine the fair market value of his or her work.

Data sets exist that indicate what the going rate is for clinicians according to specialty and geographic area. Such data are also usually related to productivity measures such as the number of patient encounters or billed revenue. Once again, the clinician must have a fair degree of confidence that the data are indeed representative of the work he or she performs. If not, the clinician must be prepared to refute such data when presented with it as a basis for determining salary or work expectations.

Data gathering may be tedious work, and the busy clinician may have little interest in statistics, contractual allowances, or practice expenses. Despite the unattractive nature of statistical analysis, the process is essential to the successful clinician. Knowing the numbers empowers the clinician to negotiate better contracts, improve quality of care, and become a more productive contributor to a practice or organization. If data are not compiled, analyzed, and presented to the right audience, the work of the clinician remains one of the organization's best kept secrets.

CHAPTER 13

THERE'S NO BUSINESS LIKE GOOD BUSINESS

When one thinks of business, especially good business, one naturally thinks of money, financial success, and profits. Hopefully, the reader has by now realized that there is more to business than generating revenue. However, it is indeed likely that generating revenue or making a living is of paramount concern to most professionals. This chapter will discuss the rules for receiving reimbursement, including the basic concepts of billing and coding. If the clinician is more philanthropic in his or her professional endeavors and not at all concerned with profit, he or she should read on anyway. Mastering the concepts of correct billing and coding will optimize revenue, but it is also *the law.*

THE RULES

There are five basic rules for reimbursement for the provision of healthcare services. Payors will pay for services that are:

1. Provided by a qualified provider
2. Included in the covered benefits
3. Medically necessary
4. Documented in the medical record
5. Coded correctly

These rules are enforced according to federal and state law. Individual insurance companies may adopt rules and regulations of their own as well.

Federal Law

The end of the Cold War in Europe put many US federal agents out of work. As in other industries in which workers become obsolete, restructuring of some federal programs resulted in the retraining of agents to investigate

Medicare and Medicaid fraud! The government did not bother to send these agents to medical school, but merely trained them to investigate potential insurance fraud through the review of medical records. Additionally, the federal government has enlisted the aid of another important group to assist in policing the billing practices of clinicians—*your patients*. The government offers incentives to patients (called whistle-blowers) for reporting what they perceive as illegal billing practices. For these reasons alone, the clinician must be informed and accurate when it comes to billing for services.

Another obviously important motivator for learning how to bill appropriately is the fact that insurance companies depend on information supplied by the clinician to process a claim and authorize payment. This requires that the clinician learn the language of the insurance industry that translates clinical work into a bill and eventually compensation. Some clinicians would argue that hiring a billing specialist or billing service to generate claims is all that is necessary to comply with regulations. Employing knowledgeable billing staff is probably a wise investment; however, unless the clinician is planning on having the billing staff in each exam room with him or her while rendering care, it is still necessary to learn proper billing rules.

There are many rules that define legal billing practice. The federal government, through the Center for Medicare and Medicaid Services (CMS), oversees Medicare and Medicaid billing. Each clinician should become familiar with the CMS rules and regulations that pertain specifically to the clinician and his or her profession.

Medicare recipients may receive care from nonphysicians, but currently payment for these services is less than the physician payment. There is no formula for determining the percentage of payment allowed a nonphysician, and many of the rules that determine payment to clinicians are more than two decades old. Logically, if payment were based on the Resource-Based Relative Value Scale, which determines payment for services based on the work effort of the provider, the cost of providing the service, and the liability or risk associated with the provision of the service, a more accurate method of determining payment could be employed (see Chapter 14).

The clinician may contract with a Medicare **managed care** program to provide care to the enrollees of such programs. The contract specifies the amount of reimbursement for services, which does not have to comply with the reimbursement schedule defined in traditional *straight* Medicare plans. Thus the clinician is able to receive more equitable reimbursement when caring for Medicare recipients covered in managed care plans.

State Law

Individual states also determine how the clinician will practice by defining scope of practice, the relationship with a physician, and prescriptive authority. Within these rules and regulations are the parameters that determine legal billing practice. States have the ability to pass laws that allow or even mandate third-party reimbursement to clinicians as long as they practice within the boundaries as defined by state law.

Individual states also have rules regarding billing for Medicaid. Many states also have a Medicaid managed care product. Rules and regulations that exist within these programs vary from state to state, and the clinician is advised to become familiar with them as they apply to the his or her practice.

Credentialing

Once the clinician is familiar with how their scope of practice is defined by the federal and state governments, he or she must become **credentialed** with government programs, managed care organizations, and third-party payors (insurance companies) in order to bill these entities and receive compensation from them. The credentialing process can be very lengthy and tedious, but similar documentation is required by each credentialing body, so once the information is assembled, it is simply a matter of duplicating it.

The clinician may be faced with three payment scenarios: payors who credential and reimburse the clinician at 100% of the physician rate, payors who reimburse the clinician at a fraction of the physician rate, and payors who cannot or will not credential nonphysician providers. (Some clinicians are mentioned in federal mandates that assure participation in government programs and others have successfully lobbied for and won mandates for third-party reimbursement in their states.) In some programs, it may be illegal for the payor to deny participation in the program to a clinician based solely on the clinician's licensure. Because the system is so convoluted, the clinician must examine all the rules so as to speak and act knowledgeably when submitting applications for credentialing.

Once the clinician determines the rules, he or she should develop an action plan that may simply involve filling out applications for the companies with whom the clinician plans to participate. When payors refuse to credential a nonphysician provider, the clinician has two options. As a first option, the clinician can offer to assist the payor with developing a credentialing mechanism for nonphysician providers. Often companies do not credential nonphysician providers because such a mechanism does not exist within the company, but with some guidance, most are willing to develop a process. The second option is to consider billing incident to a physician.

"Incident to" Billing

Many clinicians are dependent on the licensure of their collaborating physician for their legal basis for practice and must bill in the physician's name for services provided by the clinician. Other clinicians are forced to bill in the name of their collaborating physician because insurance companies do not have a mechanism for credentialing them despite laws that allow clinicians to bill for services. Additionally, when a payor reimburses a clinician at a fraction of the physician's rate, the clinician or his or her practice may choose to bill in the name of the physician.

The CMS allows a clinician to bill **incident to** a physician when providing services to Medicare recipients so long as the following rules are followed:

- The physician must see all new patients for their initial visit.
- The physician must document subsequent visits and address all new problems.
- The physician must personally supervise the clinician.
- The physician *does not* need to be consulted at each visit or co-sign each chart entry.
- The physician *must be physically present* in the office suite when the clinician is providing a service.

These rules apply to Medicare only, but Medicaid and other payors can adopt these same rules. Managed care organizations and other insurance companies can set their own rules for billing incident to a physician. These individual incident to arrangements should be made in collaboration with the clinician. If the clinician plans to bill incident to a physician, the insurance company should be notified of the arrangement and a copy of the collaborative agreements submitted with the application for credentialing. A letter defining incident to as it applies to the clinician's practice should accompany the application as well.

Fraud

Failure to bill for services according to the rules and regulations results in fraudulent billing, which is punishable by fine and/or imprisonment. The healthcare provider is responsible for all bills generated in his or her name and will be held accountable for billing done on his or her behalf. The Office of the Inspector General is responsible for investigating billing fraud.

Managed Care

Many patients are participants in managed care health plans. In efforts to control costs, patients are assigned to a primary care provider or gate keeper. The patient sees this provider for all healthcare needs and may access a specialty provider after obtaining a **referral** from the primary care provider. If the clinician provides care in a specialty office, he or she must be aware of the rules pertaining to this arrangement and work within those rules so that the patient does not incur out-of-pocket expenses for the visit.

A proactive approach to this problem is to confirm the patient's type of insurance and explanation of benefits at the time the appointment is made. With some plans, patients may self-select certain services, such as an annual well-woman exam, from their provider of choice. If the clinician detects a problem and wishes to consult another healthcare provider, the patient may have to return to his or her primary care provider to obtain this referral.

Clinicians providing care to pregnant patients may, under the rules of the insurance plan, automatically become the primary care provider for the duration of the pregnancy or they may have to defer problems unrelated to the pregnancy back to the primary provider.

The rules for reimbursement are very confusing and convoluted. It behooves the clinician to learn these rules to avoid the frustration associated with this confusion.

THE BILLING AND CODING LANGUAGE

As mentioned earlier, the process of billing and coding translates clinical work into a language that is understood by insurance companies and results in payment. Why is it imperative that the clinician learn this language?

- Compliance issues. The clinician is responsible for the bill.
- Reimbursement. Proper billing and coding enhances the reimbursement a clinician receives for services provided.
- Knowledge. The clinician has exclusive knowledge of what goes on in the examination room, delivery room, operating room, and other care areas.

Current Procedural Terminology

Each clinical service has a corresponding numeric code that describes the services provided by the clinician. Stated another way, the five-digit **Current Procedural Terminology (CPT)** code describes what service is provided and how much the clinician is to be paid. There are over 7500 CPT codes. CPT codes are divided into six sections: evaluation and management, radiology, pathology and laboratory, surgery, medicine, and anesthesia.

The sheer numbers of these codes may initially intimidate the average clinician; however, most clinicians rapidly become familiar with the most frequently used codes. Because codes are grouped by clinical specialty areas, finding the correct CPT code is easier than one might presume. CPT codes are updated annually, therefore a current CPT resource (published by the American Medical Association) is a necessity. Some specialty areas publish abbreviated resources that are specific to a particular clinical area. The clinician can contact national organizations to inquire if such references are available.

Modifiers

The uniqueness of each clinical situation does not always allow a CPT code to accurately reflect the service performed. For this reason, CPT coding includes suffixes called **modifiers** that can be added to a code for further clarification. A list of modifiers and their definitions is listed in Appendix A of CPT coding books. Modifiers denote when compensation for a service may be altered due to extenuating circumstances. Modifiers may increase or decrease reimbursement depending on their meaning. An example on the use of modifiers clarifies this point.

A patient presents after hours to the hospital with a complaint of decreased fetal movement. An external fetal monitor is applied and the nurse-midwife comes to evaluate the monitor tracing. The procedure that is billed is a fetal non-stress test and has a corresponding CPT code of 59025. The non-stress test is a procedure that contains both a technical and a professional component. The hospital will bill for the technical component and the midwife will bill for the interpretation of the test, or the professional component. The correct code in this instance is 59025-26. The modifier -26 indicates that reduced payment is indicated because the midwife interpreted the test, but did not own the equipment used for the test, nor did he or she employ the nurse who administered the test.

Conversely, had the test been performed during office hours in the clinician's office suite, no modifier would have been used because the practice could expect full payment for the procedure because the practice owned the equipment, employed the staff member administering the test, and one of the healthcare providers interpreted the test.

A scenario such as this one is straightforward, however, in some cases documentation that supports why a modifier was added may be required. A -21 modifier may be added when a service provided takes longer than what is considered reasonable. The clinician must document the time spent face-to-face with the patient when performing the procedure or service and explain why additional time was necessary.

A commonly used modifier is the -25 modifier. This suffix is used when two *separate and significant* services are performed on the same day by the same healthcare provider. For example, a physician's assistant is scheduled to perform an annual checkup on a patient who also complains of an upper-respiratory infection. The clinician can bill for the preventative medicine examination and an **evaluation and management** service that represents the additional work done to diagnose and treat the patient's other complaint. The -25 modifier is attached to the lesser of the two codes, which in this case is the evaluation and management service. The attachment of the modifier tells the insurance company that two services were performed during one visit. Reduced compensation for the evaluation and management component of the visit is reasonable because the patient made only one appointment, used one exam room, and much of the history and physical overlapped. Documentation for this visit must clearly indicate the separate work that was involved in diagnosing and treating the upper-respiratory infection. The clinician should not expect additional reimbursement for work that is already part of the routine annual physical exam.

Some insurance companies do not reimburse a clinician for two services on the same day, despite correct use of the -25 modifier. In such cases, the clinician has the following options:

- Perform both services and bill only for the preventative medicine visit but add a -22 modifier (unusual procedure or service) to the visit to denote the additional service performed.
- Treat the upper-respiratory infection and reschedule the preventative medicine visit, thus billing both separately.

Other modifiers exist to assist the clinician in relaying to the insurance company information about a service performed. The clinician must become familiar with these modifiers to ensure accurate billing.

Establishing Medical Necessity

International Classification of Diseases. Whereas CPT codes determine the clinician's level of payment, the *International Classification of Diseases,* 9th revision (ICD-9) codes determine *if* the clinician is paid. (The 10th revision of ICD codes is expected to be published by 2004.) The ICD-9 codes establish the **medical necessity** for a service by describing a diagnosis, symptom, complaint, condition, or problem. The Center for Disease Control in Atlanta, Georgia, uses ICD-9 codes for the collection of health statistics and clinical data.

When billing for services, each CPT code must be paired with at least one ICD-9 code that establishes the reason for the service. More than one ICD-9 code per CPT code is permitted if indicated. When codes are listed on a claim form for billing purposes, the most acute or immediate reason for the most extensive, invasive, or expensive procedure performed is listed first. Payment for subsequent codes is usually discounted, thus the reason for listing codes in descending order.

V Codes. Many of the services provided by a clinician are for reasons other than an injury or disease. Such visits include annual wellness examinations or visits for counseling. **V codes** are found in ICD-9. A common V code is V22—single intrauterine pregnancy.

J Codes. **J codes** are used to bill for a material or device such as an immunization or an intrauterine device.

To identify the correct ICD-9 code, the clinician uses the alphabetic index found in volume 2 of the ICD-9 book (located in the front) to locate the condition or disease. The condition, symptom, or complaint will have a corresponding three-digit number that is used to locate the condition in the tabular index (volume 1) found at the back of the ICD-9 book. From there, additional numbers following a decimal point after the three-digit number add further specificity to the diagnosis. The clinician should provide as much information as possible to the billing clerk so that the most specific code possible is noted on the claim form. Nonspecific codes may result in lower or denied payment.

ICD-9 does not include codes for *possible, probable,* or *rule out* diagnoses. In such cases where the diagnosis is not clear, the symptom or complaint is coded. Again, specificity is the key to optimizing payment.

Evaluation and Management Codes

The vast majority of services billed by clinicians are billed as office or out-patient visits. These visits are billed as level visits (levels 1–5) based on the amount of history, physical exam, and medical decision making involved in the visit.

History. The history component includes the chief complaint, or reason for the visit, a history of the present illness, a review of systems, and the patient's past medical history, family history, and social history. Four levels of history are included in evaluation and management coding: a problem focused history, an expanded problem focused history, a detailed history, and a comprehensive history.

Problem Focused History. A problem focused history includes:

- The chief complaint
- A brief history of the present illness (one to three elements) (Elements of the history of the present illness include: location, duration, severity, intensity, and exacerbating or alleviating factors of the chief complaint).
- No review of systems or past, family, or social history is required.

Expanded Problem Focused History. An expanded problem focused history includes:

- The chief complaint
- A brief history of the present illness (one to three elements)
- A problem-pertinent review of systems
- No past, family, or social history

Detailed History. A detailed history includes:

- The chief complaint
- An extended history of the present illness (at least four elements)
- An extended review of systems (two to nine systems)
- A pertinent past, family, or social history

Comprehensive History. A comprehensive history includes:

- The chief complaint
- An extended history of the present illness
- A complete review of systems (10 or more systems)
- A complete past, family and social history (All three components of past, family, and social history are required when providing services to a new patient, whereas two of three components are required for an established patient.)

Physical Examination. Similar to history, evaluation and management codes include four levels of physical examination, including a problem focused exam, an expanded problem focused exam, a detailed exam, and a comprehensive exam. For the purposes of the physical examination, body areas or systems are evaluated.

Body systems include:

- Head, including the face
- Neck
- Chest, including the breasts and axilla
- Abdomen
- Genitalia, groin, and buttocks
- Back, including the spine
- Each extremity

Organ systems include:

- Opthalmologic
- Otolaryngologic
- Cardiovascular
- Respiratory
- Endocrine
- Gastrointestinal
- Genitourinary
- Musculoskeletal
- Integumentary
- Neurologic
- Psychiatric
- Hematologic/lymphatic
- Allergic/immunologic

Also included is a constitutional exam, which includes vital signs and comments about the patient's general appearance. Three constitutional findings are comparable to one body area or organ system.

Currently, the clinician may choose to document the physical exam using either the 1995 or 1997 federal guidelines. Guidelines developed in 2000 have been proposed, but as of fall 2003, have yet to be implemented. The clinician is advised to examine current law when documenting the physical exam. For purposes of illustration, this chapter will use the 1995 guidelines.

Problem Focused Exam. The affected organ system is examined.

Expanded Problem Focused Exam. The affected organ system is examined. A limited exam of two to four symptomatic or related organ systems also are examined.

Detailed Exam. The affected system plus five to seven other systems are examined.

Comprehensive Exam. The affected organ system plus 8 to 12 other systems are examined.

A variety of resources offer chart forms that assist the clinician with documenting a physical examination. Many were developed in order to allow for compliance with federal documentation guidelines. Some auditors advise that it is acceptable for a clinician to circle or check "normal" when performing an examination, but it is unacceptable to run a single line down through the "normal" boxes. Each element must be checked individually.

Elements of Medical Decision Making. Four levels of medical decision making are included in evaluation and management coding: straightforward, low complexity, moderate complexity, and high complexity. To determine the level of medical decision making, the clinician must consider three elements:

1. The number of diagnoses or management options to consider, including:
    - Number and types of problems addressed
    - Complexity of establishing a diagnosis
    - Number of management decisions made
2. The amount and complexity of data to be obtained, reviewed, or analyzed, including:
    - Types or amount of testing ordered
    - Obtaining old medical records
    - Obtaining a history from someone other than the patient
    - Discussing results of tests with the provider who performed the test
    - Personally reviewing an image, tracing, or specimen
3. The risk of complications, morbidity, or mortality associated with:
    - The presenting problem
    - Diagnostic procedures
    - Management options

To determine the level of medical decision making, all three elements are considered, and each level is assigned a rating of minimal, limited, moderate, or high complexity. The highest two of the three elements determine the level of medical decision making.

For example, a patient who presents with a limited number of diagnoses and management options who requires a moderate amount of testing or data review and has limited risk of morbidity would require low-complexity medical decision making.

As an additional example, a patient presenting with a moderate number of potential diagnoses who requires a high amount of data be reviewed and is at high risk for morbidity or mortality would require high-complexity medical decision making.

Selecting an Evaluation and Management Level. To determine the level of evaluation and management, the clinician determines:

- The level of medical decision making
- The type of history taken
- The type of physical examination performed
- If the patient is an *established* or *new* patient

A *new* patient is one who has not been seen by anyone of the same specialty in the clinician's group for 3 years. "Services" include face-to-face services that were submitted for reimbursement such as blood tests or other billed services. Services that are not included are telephone contacts or prescription renewals. Thus, if no billable services are provided in a period of 3 years, an *old* patient becomes a *new* patient for billing purposes.

An *established* patient includes patients that may have followed a new provider to the practice from another practice. Even if the patient is unknown to the other providers in the practice, he or she is still considered an established patient in the practice.

Once it has been determined if the patient is a new or established patient, Tables 13.1 and 13.2 are used to determine the evaluation and management level visit.

To assign a level visit to a new patient encounter, select the highest level documented by all three elements (history, physical exam, and medical decision making). The times offered are guidelines, but the clinician only bills based on the amount of time the encounter took if more than 50% of the visit involved counseling, teaching, or advising the patient.

TABLE 13.1 EVALUATION AND MANAGEMENT LEVEL VISITS (NEW PATIENTS)

Code	History	Exam	Decision Making	Time (minutes)
99201	Problem focused	Problem focused	Straightforward	10
99202	Expanded problem focused	Expanded problem focused	Straightforward	20
99203	Detailed	Detailed	Low	30
99204	Comprehensive	Comprehensive	Moderate	45
99205	Comprehensive	Comprehensive	High	60

TABLE 13.2 EVALUATION AND MANAGEMENT LEVEL VISITS (ESTABLISHED PATIENTS)

Code	History	Exam	Decision Making	Time (minutes)
99211				5
99212	Problem focused	Problem focused	Straightforward	10
99213	Expanded problem focused	Expanded problem focused	Low	15
99214	Detailed	Detailed	Moderate	25
99215	Comprehensive	Comprehensive	High	40

To assign a level visit to an established patient encounter, select the highest level documented by two of the three elements (history, physical exam, and medical decision making). Again, the times offered are guidelines, but the clinician only bills based on the amount of time the encounter took if more than 50% of the visit involved counseling, teaching, or advising the patient.

Counseling

At times, a clinician sees a patient for the purpose of providing education or counseling or to discuss test results. Such visits do not include a physical exam and are billed based on the time the clinician spends face-to-face with the patient. The evaluation and management tables for new and established patients are used to select a level visit based on time.

Preventative Medicine Visits

With today's focus on wellness, many patients present annually for **preventative medicine visits** for the purposes of screening and risk-factor reduction. Preventative medicine visits are coded according to the patient's age and are separated into categories of new and established patients.

Such visits include:

- A comprehensive history
- A comprehensive physical exam
- Counseling, anticipatory guidance, and risk-factor reduction
- Age-appropriate laboratory testing and/or diagnostic procedures

As discussed earlier, the patient may present for an annual preventative medicine visit and also complain of one or more problems at this visit. The clinician has the option of addressing the problem and rescheduling the wellness exam, providing both services and adding a -22 modifier onto the code for the preventative medicine visit, or billing both services. When billing both services, the portion of the visit that is separate and specific to the problem addressed is documented and the appropriate evaluation and management level visit is selected and billed in addition to the preventative medicine visit. The evaluation and management level visit would have a -25 modifier attached.

Consults and Referrals

It is common for the clinician to seek the opinion of another healthcare provider when faced with complications or problems beyond the scope of practice of the clinician. A **consult** differs from a referral in the following ways:

- A problem is suspected but not known
- An opinion or advice is sought rather than transfer of care
- A written request for advice is made (consult)
- A written opinion is returned to the clinician (consult)

Healthcare providers who provide consultations are required to perform and document a history, an examination, and medical decision making. Consultation codes (99241–99245) reimburse at higher levels than evaluation and management visits. When addressing a letter requesting the opinion of a healthcare provider, the clinician is advised to *request the opinion* of the healthcare provider or ask the provider to *please evaluate* the patient. If the letter states that the clinician is *referring* the patient for a suspected problem, an auditor may be confused as to whether this visit was a consultation or a referral. If the healthcare provider retains the patient for further management of a problem, the first visit is billed as a consultation and subsequent visits are billed as evaluation and management visits based on the level of history, examination, and medical decision making involved in the visit.

Global Charges

Insurance companies may lump charges for some services together into global charges. This is done for services that have an established amount of work involved that universally applies to the majority of patients. Global charges exist for obstetric care that includes routine ante-, intra-, and postpartum care. Global charges also exist for surgical procedures that include the routine pre- and postoperative care that is commonly provided. The CPT code book describes what is included in these packages. The clinician is permitted to submit additional charges when services are provided in addition to what is covered in the global package.

BILLING MODELS

Many billing models exist in which the clinician bills for and expects reimbursement. Some clinicians bill independently under their own provider numbers. Some bill incident to a physician. Others submit bills under a practice identification number. Each model has various benefits and drawbacks. Benefits of such models include the retention of independence and control. Drawbacks, depending on the model, include the assumption of financial risk, a lack of security, and potential fraud. The clinician presented with the option of choosing a billing model is advised to evaluate all of the options available and select the model that works best for him or her.

VARIABLES AFFECTING REIMBURSEMENT

At the beginning of this chapter, five criteria for receiving payment from a payor were listed. The variables that affect reimbursement involve those five criteria. Services must be:

1. Provided by a qualified provider
    - Credential providers with the payor
    - Follow incident to rules
    - Determine who is the primary care provider
2. Included in the covered benefits
    - Evaluate benefits prior to scheduling an appointment
    - Determine the services that are approved
    - Obtain a referral if necessary
    - Determine if preauthorization is required
    - Determine services included and excluded in global packages
3. Medically necessary
    - Establish medical necessity
4. Documented correctly
    - Ensure that documentation supports the level of service billed
    - Ensure the documentation matches the diagnosis
    - Avoid incomplete or illegible documentation
5. Coded correctly
    - Avoid using nonspecific codes
    - Use the correct codes
    - Do not omit codes
    - Use modifiers when indicated

ENHANCING REIMBURSEMENT

Reimbursement is enhanced when the clinician and the practice follow these five rules. Additionally, it is the practice's responsibility to use the correct forms when submitting a bill and to bill frequently and accurately. If a co-pay is required of the patient for outpatient services, this should be collected at the time of service.

Someone in the practice should be responsible for monitoring the accounts receivable and determine how long it takes to get paid for a service. Seventy percent of a practice's accounts receivable should be received in 90 days or less. Accounts that are aged more than 90 days are less likely to be paid.

A financially savvy practice conducts regular audits to ensure that all healthcare providers in the practice are documenting and coding accurately. Encounter forms should be revised periodically to reflect coding changes, and they should be user friendly for the clinician.

Rejected or denied claims should be examined and resubmitted once corrections are made. Downgrades can result in increased reimbursement if accompanied by a letter explaining the services provided when the bill is resubmitted.

INPATIENT CHARGES

This chapter did not discuss charges that are of interest to clinicians providing services in the inpatient or emergency setting. For these clinicians, another set of billing codes apply; however, the levels are determined based on the history, physical exam, and medical decision making involved, thus employing the same principles of evaluation and management coding.

FACILITY CHARGES

Facility charges are another subset of charges with which the clinician may wish to become familiar. Facility charges include use of a hospital, surgical center, birth center, or other healthcare facility. Insurance companies usually have credentialing or licensing requirements for facilities that are necessary for the facility to receive reimbursement. The rules and regulations for the accreditation or licensing of facilities are typically found in the state's public health laws.

With respect to facility fees, one of the rules that may be of interest to the clinician is the requirement that the facility list the attending healthcare provider when submitting a claim for reimbursement. If that provider is not credentialed by the insurance company, the facility may not be able to receive reimbursement. Thus, facilities are not willing to grant admitting privileges to clinicians who are not credentialed by insurance companies or to clinicians who receive reimbursement at a discount of the physician's rate. Instead, these facilities prefer to admit patients under a collaborating physician.

Billing, coding, and getting paid involve a complex system of rules and regulations that are often unique to the individual payor. The clinician must learn the language that translates clinical services into revenue. This chapter is not intended to be a comprehensive study of billing and coding, but instead serves to introduce some of the basic concepts associated with the topics.

Because financial viability should be of paramount concern to the clinician with regards to his or her value to a practice or organization, the clinician is strongly advised to continue his or her study of billing and coding, particularly because each clinical specialty area has its own nuances specific to the specialty.

The clinician is also cautioned to make the study of billing and coding an ongoing process because codes are frequently updated to reflect current practice trends and the rules with regards to billing and coding are constantly being revised. Staying current with respect to billing and coding requires the same amount of effort as keeping up with changes in clinical practice. The business savvy clinician will devote time and attention to accurate billing and coding.

CHAPTER 14

WORTH YOUR WEIGHT IN GOLD

Historically, nonphysician clinicians were used in medically underserved or inner-city areas—places where the recruitment and retention of physicians was nearly impossible. The clinician practicing in such situations was at liberty to provide care without a great deal of scrutiny, especially when it came to business issues, productivity, and generating revenue. Most of the clientele were either poor, covered by public aid, undocumented aliens, or minorities. The clinicians worked in programs that were grant funded or charity sponsored or in public health centers. Clinicians practicing in such environments often dealt with a lack of equipment, poor resources, and little support staff. Their primary concern was to provide health care. No one worried too much about billing, revenue, and productivity.

The clinician working in a clinic or hospital-owned service collected a paycheck without much thought to individual productivity, profit sharing, or the bottom line. Clinicians in a private practice, to some extent, were held more accountable for their share of the work, but in general, most did not know the first thing about accounting for one's financial contributions to a practice. These clinicians had the luxury of focusing on the quality of care they provided without worrying too much about quantity.

PRODUCTIVITY DATA SETS

In today's competitive healthcare environment, fiscal responsibility and productivity are now at the forefront. Even those clinicians that work for large institutions are evaluated and often compensated based on some formula that measures productivity. The **Medical Group Management Association (MGMA)** collects data from organizations that are its members describing productivity in a variety of venues, including outpatient visits or billed revenue. The data are compiled according to geographic region and published annually. Data are presented as quartiles of productivity.

Although such data are helpful in establishing benchmarks for productivity, one must be cautious about placing all of his or her eggs in one basket. The data generated by MGMA are collected via a complex questionnaire that is most likely completed by administrators. Very few clinicians have had the opportunity to complete or even have input into the completion of such a questionnaire. In fact, very few practicing clinicians would have sufficient knowledge to accurately answer the questions asked.

Another fault of the data compiled by MGMA is that the sample size of clinicians who are not physicians is often small. MGMA only samples its members, thus the data may or may not be from an adequate sample that is representative of clinical practice.

A further problem with any data set that attempts to be representative of the practice of clinicians who are not physicians is that, as pointed out in previous chapters, the practice of clinicians varies widely and is dependent on state laws, local rules and regulations, and individual practice patterns. One can easily find two clinicians with similar educational background and specialty area working in the same city with completely different practice patterns.

This does not mean clinicians can dodge the issue of productivity. What it does mean is that they must understand how they are being evaluated and consider the variety of tools used to quantify productivity. Some of the more common methods will be discussed here.

PATIENT ENCOUNTERS

One of the easiest methods to determine the productivity of a healthcare provider is to count numbers of patients seen in the office over a specified time period. The term used in this case is **patient encounters** or **outpatient visits.** This is a very simple way of quantifying workload. Data can be generated by a computer using billing records or patient schedule sheets. If all providers see the same type of patients, such a system is very easy to implement.

However, most clinicians know that all patient encounters do not take the same amount of time, nor do they require the same amount of work or skill from the clinician. Visits for procedures or other lengthy services may take more time and produce more revenue, but still count as one encounter with this system. If a clinician is scheduled to perform a procedure that takes 45 minutes, he or she will be credited with one encounter, whereas a colleague may see three patients with less acute problems in the same 45 minutes and receive credit for three encounters. In areas where no-shows for appointments are high, the clinician who has a scheduled procedure loses the opportunity to count that visit if the patient fails to show for the appointment. The clinician then has 45 minutes of downtime on his or her schedule. Similarly, clinicians working in new or developing office sites where the patient schedule is not yet full are penalized when evaluation of productivity is based on visits.

Another difficulty with this method of measurement is that it does not account for work done outside of the office setting. Clinicians who assist with surgery or perform other inpatient services find that a significant proportion of their workload is unaccounted for. Clinicians who work in such settings are usually responsible for being available after hours, during nights, holidays, and weekends. Evaluating productivity according to "visits" does not recognize the acute nature of inpatient or after-hours care, nor does it account for or reward a clinician for the demands and sacrifices made when working a nontraditional schedule.

In some instances, it may be helpful to count visits or to quantify certain services. For instance, a midwifery service may want to look at how many births per midwife are attended annually. Again, many variables may be considered in such a measurement, such as the proportion of obstetric patients in a women's health service. One midwifery service may see only obstetric patients, whereas another may have a 30% gynecologic patient load, plus have some teaching responsibilities as a faculty for a university midwifery or medical school education program. These cases illustrate how difficult it is to apply a single measurement to all practices equitably.

BILLED REVENUE

Another method of evaluating productivity is by evaluating **billed revenue.** Revenue is generated when a service is provided. Clinicians in similar practice settings and specialty areas should be expected to generate comparable revenue. In our society, dollars and cents speak loudly, thus work that is translated into dollars is highly reflective of a clinician's value to a practice or organization. Revenue is easy to count and easy to compare with another clinician.

As with patient visits, there are problems with evaluating a clinician by billed revenue. First, and most importantly, as we have learned before, most bills for services are not generated in the name of the nonphysician clinician. Because insurance companies fail to universally credential all clinicians, practices are forced to bill under the physician for a majority of services rendered. Unless an internal mechanism for allocating revenue to the nonphysician is developed, the amount of billed revenue that is generated by the clinician is often difficult to document accurately. If these internal mechanisms do exist, the clinician must have confidence in the record-keeping system that accounts for his or her work.

Other problems exist with collecting data on billed revenue. When services are billed globally, meaning several services are lumped together into one charge, as with the prenatal care, delivery, and postpartum package, dividing the global charge among several providers may prove difficult. It is unrealistic to expect anyone to break up the individual components of such services for the purpose of allocating billed revenue.

Another issue of compensation formulas based on billed revenue is the possibility of "padding the numbers" with unnecessary procedures. Many mechanisms exist today that force a provider to justify the medical necessity of all medical services provided. However, despite all the checks and balances, a healthcare provider who has billed revenue as an incentive to be productive must be monitored for quality as well.

RESOURCE-BASED RELATIVE VALUE UNITS

A new method of evaluating productivity is rapidly gaining acceptance in the healthcare business. Based on a system developed at Harvard in the 1980s, the **Resource-Based Relative Value Scale (RBRVS)** is an innovative method developed to measure the cost of providing a service while creating equity in physician reimbursement across clinical specialties.[1] This method was adopted by the HCFA in 1992 to determine Medicare payments. **Relative Value Units (RVUs)** began to be used to measure healthcare productivity in the late 1990s.

The system uses a formula that considers the work effort of the provider, the resources required to provide the service, and the liability associated with the provision of the service. The service is then assigned a number of RVUs based on this formula. Many CPT codes have RVUs assigned to them. The RVUs are modified somewhat to take regional or geographical differences into consideration. Global charges are assigned RVUs, but the total RVU package may be broken down and allocated to specific components of the global service.

The RVU system allows for a systematic, measurable accounting of the work done by each healthcare provider. Assigning RVUs to nonclinical activities, such as teaching classes or administrative duties, is an optional way of including this type of work into total productivity. In developing practices or satellite clinics, a minimum number of RVUs for staffing such a site may be offered so as not to penalize the clinician who is assigned to the site with a lower volume of patients or procedures.

However, measuring productivity by RVUs has its disadvantages. RVUs do not measure coordination of care or other efforts of the care provider not directly related to patient contact. Not all CPT codes have been assigned RVUs, and some specialties argue that the codes assigned to their common procedures are too low.

RVUs do not account for the differences in quality of care either. They do not take into account the needs of different patient populations, the experience of the clinician, or the amount of support services available to assist with care delivery. Of perhaps most interest to the clinician is the fact that RVUs were developed to measure *physician* work, and because all clinicians do not work the same way as physicians do, using RVUs to evaluate nonphysicians may be inaccurate.

Because the use of RVUs is fairly recent, not all practices are generating data on RVUs, but the method is gaining in popularity. The savvy clinician should become familiar with the RBRVS system. If compensation is to occur based on RVUs, a clinician should have the opportunity to evaluate a year's worth of data before determining an acceptable goal for productivity. Because few clinicians are aware of what their RVU-earning capacity is, contracting to be compensated based on RVUs without some idea of what this translates to in terms of workload would be like signing a blank check.

PRODUCTIVITY-BASED CONTRACTS

A provider in private practice is motivated to be productive based on the need to cover practice expenses and maintain the service, as well as to generate personal income. The employed healthcare provider may lapse into complacency in a situation in which he or she is not directly responsible for expenses nor held responsible for the practice's budget. Thus, in an attempt to provide incentives to providers in this situation, productivity-based contracts have been developed. Productivity-based contracts calculate the clinician's compensation package based on a formula that measures productivity. Although the measuring of productivity is in most cases inevitable, the clinician must exercise caution when such measures are applied to an individual or practice.

In situations where nonphysician providers practice with physicians in the same practice, one is cautioned to ensure that the collaborative nature of the practice is not compromised by the development of a productivity-based system. One way to accomplish this is to avoid measuring all the providers (physicians and clinicians) by the same yardstick. The yardstick is only so long, or stated another way, no matter how many slices, a pie is only so big. Thus, consider evaluating the physicians by one method (billed revenue) and the other clinicians by another (RVUs), for example.

Competition can also exist within a group of like clinicians. Consider pooling contributions to productivity in cases in which there is confidence that each clinician is doing his or her share of the work. This is most useful in situations in which the individual clinicians have little control over the opportunity to be productive (staffing a labor and delivery unit or emergency room) or clinicians within the group each possess specialty skills that contribute to the overall productivity of the group, but productivity is allocated disproportionately. For example, the clinician who possesses a specialty skill that has more RVUs assigned or produces more revenue may provide this service to 10 patients in a clinic session. Another clinician may provide a more routine service to 20 clients in the same session. Is one clinician more valuable than another? Both are contributing to the needs of the patients served by the practice. Exercise caution so that productivity measures do not erode the collegial relationship between clinicians.

For purposes of contracting, one must evaluate the formulas for productivity measurement and select that method that most closely represents the work done by the clinician. However, it is possible to keep statistics on multiple measures. This is helpful in explaining why one clinician may be an outlier when compared to others in the same group.

For instance, a nurse practitioner in an OB/GYN office accumulated significantly fewer RVUs than the other nurse practitioners in the same office. RVUs assigned to gynecologic services are notoriously low when compared to other services, but charges for gynecologic services are typically better than for obstetric services. Thus, when the nurse practitioner's billed revenue was compared to that of her colleagues, she had significantly outperformed them.

Whatever the measure employed, the clinician should have confidence in the methods used to compute the productivity, and he or she should believe that the method used most accurately reflects all work that is done. Efforts to account for value that is not related to the generation of revenue should be examined. Most importantly, in efforts to demonstrate productivity, quality should never be compromised for quantity.

The measurement of productivity and contracts that compensate based on productivity are inevitable. When salary is determined based on productivity, the clinician should consider negotiating a base salary that ensures an adequate income for living expenses with bonuses paid at agreed upon intervals based on productivity. This way, in cases of peaks and valleys or fluctuations in patient volume, the clinician is able to feel somewhat secure. In private practice, in which the healthcare providers metaphorically "eat what they kill," budgeting for a base salary as a part of the practice's expenses is wise. Revenue above expenses is then shared between providers on a regular basis as appropriate.

Measuring work either formally or informally will affect each clinician at some point in his or her career. Understanding the implications and the methods used to evaluate productivity should be a basic part of every clinician's practice. Whenever possible, a combination of methods should be used when evaluating productivity. As more data are generated by clinicians other than physicians, better and more applicable statistics will be available.

NOTE

1. RBRVS: Slowly Bleeding Your Practice Dry: Rake Report, http://leaton/cole.com/rake2.pdf (August 28, 2000).

CHAPTER 15

THERE'S SAFETY IN NUMBERS

In previous chapters, the clinician has been advised, for various reasons, to contact the local or national organization that represents the clinician's practice or profession. Several organizations exist whose membership is composed of clinicians who share similar educational preparation, licensure, and scope of practice. The ultimate purpose of these organizations is to provide a structure that supports the individual clinician, as well as the profession as a whole.

In graduate education programs, courses that address professional development often introduce the student to the organization that represents his or her particular clinical area of practice or profession. Membership in such an organization should be considered a professional obligation, and the benefits of membership are many.

Most professional organizations are multifaceted and serve the profession in several areas, including:

- Establishing standards for education
- Establishing clinical standards for practice
- Coordination of research
- Political action
- Professional support
- Marketing and public relations
- Quality management
- Networking

ESTABLISHING STANDARDS FOR EDUCATION

Education Programs

The national organization may assist with curriculum development in the programs that prepare the clinician for practice or develop a list of **core**

compentencies that must be included in all education programs. These programs may receive preaccreditation from the national organization and become fully accredited after demonstrating the ability to adequately prepare clinicians for practice. Maintenance of accreditation is the responsibility of the education program, and the program's accreditation is evaluated periodically by the national accrediting organization.

Continuing Education

The national organization will describe the continuing education requirements that its members must meet to maintain clinical competence. (States may accept these requirements or impose their own rules for continuing education and maintenance of licensure within the state.) The national organization may sponsor continuing education activities in the form of conferences or modules or may grant continuing education credit to an organization or individual who completes the application process for requesting credit. The application process ensures that the content and the presenter meet the qualifications for continuing education as defined by the professional organization.

The purpose of some publications produced by the organization may be the dissemination of information to or education of the organization's members.

ESTABLISHING CLINICAL STANDARDS FOR PRACTICE

One of the most important functions of the national organization is to define the professionals whom it represents and to define the practice of those professionals. The national organization establishes clinical standards for practice, which forms the foundation for the legal basis for practice of the clinician. The organization will not explicitly define a clinician's scope of practice, because many variables define the scope of practice for the individual clinician (see Chapter 11). The organization will support a clinician's right to practice and define the core competencies in which the clinician has demonstrated proficiency through education and accreditation.

If the clinician chooses to add advanced skills to his or her repertoire, the national organization can describe the mechanism for doing so.

The organization may publish position statements or clinical bulletins for the purpose of uniting its members in policy or practice.

COORDINATION OF RESEARCH

Clinical Research

The organization may facilitate or encourage research that leads to improving care or demonstrating the competence or contributions of its professionals to health care. Such research may be published in journals produced by the organization.

Demographic Data

The organization may conduct research or survey its membership to provide descriptive data regarding its members.

POLITICAL ACTION

The national organization will often employ policy analysts that assist the membership with identifying strategic goals and legislative initiatives. The national organization usually has local chapters that stay abreast of state rules and regulations with the assistance and leadership provided by the national office. The professional organization proactively lobbies for laws that benefit clinicians or their patients by improving access to care or the quality of healthcare delivery.

The national office also serves as a resource for members as they enter the political arena by instructing them in the art of political activism.

PROFESSIONAL SUPPORT

One of the most valuable benefits of belonging to a national organization is the professional support it provides for its membership. Crisis intervention is one of the most important services provided to a clinician. Help is given in the form of practical advice, documentation, strategic planning, and legislative or legal advice.

It is often in times of crisis that some members first recognize the need of the services of the organization. However, the professional organization's value is not limited to crisis intervention. Support comes in numerous forms, including assistance with obtaining licensure or privileges, guidance with the development of practice guidelines, and resources for professional development. The organization might also help with strategy when a clinician is under attack or in danger of losing a job or help to justify a clinician's right to practice. Assistance with starting a practice and help with basic business concepts also may be provided.

The professional-support arm of the national organization often develops literature that supports the clinician and his or her practice. The organization may produce handbooks that help define clinical practice or assist the clinician with business development.

MARKETING AND PUBLIC RELATIONS

The professional organization is naturally concerned about the image of its membership, thus it devotes much time and resources to public relations.

When misinformation and prejudice are commonplace issues that present barriers to the clinicians' practice, the national organization will strive to increase public awareness and acceptance of the professionals it represents.

The organization may also assist the individual clinician with marketing and media relationships. Some organizations have developed presentations or literature that the clinician can use when preparing a presentation for the board of trustees or the local women's guild. The organization may be contacted regularly by the media to comment on news that is pertinent to the members. The public relations officer hired by the organization will monitor and disseminate to the membership news that may be of interest to the organization's members.

Educating the membership on the basics of marketing and public relations may also be a focus of the national office, because its members are the organization's ambassadors to the general public.

QUALITY MANAGEMENT

The national organization may assist its members in developing mechanisms for peer review and quality management. In doing so, the national organization can assist the membership in demonstrating clinical excellence and professional growth.

Developing national benchmarks for the profession should be a function of national organizations because current benchmarks were developed based on physician practice.

NETWORKING

Most national organizations also have regional or local offices or chapters that provide for communication between the individual clinician and the national office. These regional and local branches are composed of members who share a common profession and who want to address issues unique to a region or locality. Through membership in these local chapters, the clinician has the opportunity to develop a professional peer group that can then offer support and advice to the clinician. This is particularly important when a clinician is the sole nonphysician provider in a practice, organization, or even a city.

Networking opportunities exist for members that stretch beyond the borders of practice or even region. Through membership in an organization, members may be directed to mentors or other professionals who can serve as resources to the clinician. The national organization may also form alliances or affiliations with members of other organizations that share common interests.

The national organization may also provide the opportunity for networking on an international level when organizations with similar goals or clinical focus interact with one another.

MEMBERSHIP

Membership in a national professional organization is voluntary, but the prospective member must meet specific criteria for membership. An annual membership fee is usually required that contributes to the operations of the organization. Some clinicians may see membership in such an organization as a frivolous expense that the new clinician struggling to pay off student loans and make a living can ill afford. However, if one would consider all of the potential benefits of membership, it is the new clinician who often needs the services of the member organization the most.

MAXIMIZING YOUR BENEFITS

The premise, "you get out of it what you put into it," certainly applies to professional organizations. If a clinician chooses to neglect the opportunity to interact with other professionals of similar education and practice, remains ignorant of politics affecting practice, or shows no interest in furthering the goals or development of his or her profession, the clinician may see membership in a professional organization as unnecessary. It is the inactive member who may ask the question, "What are my dues supporting?"

Through membership in a national organization, the clinician receives newsletters or attends educational forums that serve to keep him or her up-to-date on the latest technology, legislation, or developments directly affecting the clinician and his or her practice.

Clinicians are intimately affected by local rules and regulations. The complacent clinician in a satisfying collaborative relationship may not feel the immediate need to form an alliance with a professional organization. However, clinicians are also affected by national issues such as the cost of malpractice insurance, health maintenance organizations, and capitated care. Broader issues such as insurance reimbursement and prescriptive authority also affect all nonphysician healthcare providers.

Individual clinicians may feel overwhelmed by the burden of making a living, citing the demands of private practice or long clinical hours as the reason for lack of involvement in professional groups. Some may feel handicapped by a lack of political savvy. Others may cite a lack of interest in bureaucracy as a reason for nonmembership. Although clinicians need to carefully balance all of the roles in which they participate, the budgeting of time and money must include support of the professional organization.

Admittedly, organized medicine and traditional health care has not unconditionally embraced the practice of nonphysician providers. Public ignorance continues to be an albatross around the necks of hardworking clinicians. It is through the work of organized individuals that change in policy and public opinion occurs. The professional clinician has a responsibility to support his or her national organization and its local chapters.

In addition to national organizations, clinicians will also have numerous opportunities to align themselves with other professional groups or societies. These common interest groups also focus primarily on education, politics, and peer support. The busy clinician must choose which of these groups deserve his or her support and energy. When evaluating the value of joining such organizations, ask yourself two questions:

1. *What can this group do for me?* Does the group provide the opportunity to network with others in the same or a similar profession? Does the group offer educational opportunities that may improve my clinical practice? Does the group have a political agenda that is pertinent to me?
2. *What can I do for this group?* Can I support the group with either my time or money? Do I have other resources that may benefit the group?

In summary, the benefits of membership in professional organizations are many. The goals of the national organization representing a clinician are to support, educate, and promote the practice of the membership. Clinicians are busy professionals who must budget their time and money wisely. The benefits of professional membership far outweigh the cost because, after all, there is safety in numbers.

CHAPTER 16

THE HONEYMOON NEVER LASTS

So, you have just negotiated a great contract, obtained hospital admitting privileges, or successfully lobbied to change state rules and regulations to allow independent prescriptive authority. The administrator is your advocate, the physician is your partner, and your family has stopped worrying that you are doing something illegal.

Although you may celebrate your victories or revel in your newfound security, remember that the honeymoon never lasts. Administrators, staff, physicians, and patients come and go, and the ones that stay do not remember the past for very long. Keep statistics and graphs to remind people where you have been. The ebb and flow of the tides that affect healthcare delivery will continue to present challenges and barriers to practice.

This does not mean that we live in a world filled with bogeymen, it just means the clinician should keep a vigilant eye and ear on the environment in which he or she works. In some cases, the clinician must learn to dodge the bullets that are flung his or her way with the grace of a ballet dancer. New threats will present new opportunities for the disruptive innovator.

Suggested Readings

Abood, Sheila, and David Keepnews. *Understanding Payment for APN Service.* Vol. 1–4. Washington, DC: American Nurse's Association, 2002.

American Academy of Physician's Assistants. *Contacts and Contracts.* Alexandria, VA: American Academy of Physician's Assistants, 1997.

American Academy of Physician's Assistants. *From Program to Practice.* Alexandria, VA: American Academy of Physician's Assistants, 2002.

American Academy of Physician's Assistants. *Managing Risk.* Alexandria, VA: American Academy of Physician's Assistants, 1994.

American Academy of Physician's Assistants. *PAs: State Laws and Regulations,* 9th ed. Alexandria, VA: American Academy of Physician's Assistants, 2002.

American Academy of Physician's Assistants. *PA Third-Party Coverage.* Alexandria, VA: American Academy of Physician's Assistants, 2000.

American College of Nurse Midwives. *Clinical Privileges and Credentialing Handbook.* Washington, DC: American College of Nurse Midwives, 2001.

American College of Nurse Midwives. *Getting Paid: Billing, Coding, and Payment for Nurse-Midwifery Services.* Washington, DC: American College of Nurse Midwives, 2002.

American College of Nurse Midwives. *Marketing and Public Relations Handbook.* Washington, DC: American College of Nurse Midwives, 2000.

American College of Nurse Midwives. *Minding Your Own Business: Business Plans for Midwifery Practices.* Washington DC: American College of Nurse Midwives, 2000.

American College of Nurse Midwives. *Nurse-Midwifery Today, a Handbook of State Laws and Regulations.* Washington, DC: American College of Nurse Midwives, 2002.

American College of Nurse Midwives. *Professional Liability Handbook.* Washington, DC: American College of Nurse Midwives, 2003, http://www.midwife.org/prof/.

American College of Nurse Midwives. *Strategies for Influencing State Policy-Document Set.* Washington, DC: American College of Nurse Midwives, 2002.

American College of Nurse Midwives. *Taking Action: A State Advocacy Handbook.* Washington, DC: American College of Nurse Midwives, 2003.

American Medical Association. *CPT 2003: Current Procedural Terminology.* Chicago: American Medical Association, 2002.

Bourne, Heidi. *A Great Deal! Compensation Negotiation for Nurse Practitioners and Physician's Assistants,* 4th ed. Portland, OR: Open Spaces, 2001.

Buppert, Carolyn. *Negotiating Terms of Employment.* Annapolis, MD: Law Offices of Carolyn Buppert, 2002.

Buppert, Carolyn. *Nurse Practitioner's Business Practice and Legal Guide.* Boston: Jones & Bartlett, 1999.

Carey, Raymond G., and Robert C. Lloyd. *Measuring Quality Improvement in Healthcare: A Guide to Statistical Process Control Applications.* Milwaukee, WI: American Society for Quality, 2000.

Fisher, Roger, and William Ury. *Getting Past No: Negotiating Your Way from Confrontation to Cooperation.* Riverdale, MA: Bantam Doubleday Dell Publishers, 1993.

Fisher, Roger, and William Ury. *Getting to Yes: Negotiating Agreement Without Giving In.* 2nd ed. East Rutherford, NJ: Penguin USA, 1991.

Jenkins, Susan M., "The Myth of Vicarious Liability: Impact on Barriers to Nurse-Midwifery Practice." *Journal of Nurse-Midwifery* 39(1994): 98–106.

Letz, Kevin L. *Business Essentials for Nurse Practitioners.* South Coast Metro, CA: Practice Builders, 2002.

National Association of Pediatric Nurse Associates and Practitioners. *Career Resource Kit.* http://www.napnap.org/catalog/careerresourcekit.

Partnerships for Training. *Building a Practice.* Association of Academic Health Centers. http://www.pftweb.org, 2003.

Paulson, Paulson, and John Katzman. *The Complete Idiot's Guide to Starting Your Own Business.* Hampshire, England: Alpha Books, MacMillen, 2000.

Physician ICD-9-CM: International Classification of Diseases, 9th Revision: Clinical Modification, 5th ed. Salt Lake City, UT: Medicode, 1998.

Ross, Marilyn. *Shameless Marketing for Brazen Hussies: 307 Awesome Money-Making Strategies for Savvy Entrepreneurs.* Buena Vista, CO: Communication Creativity, 2000.

Small Business Administration. *Starting Your Own Business.* http://www.sba.gov/starting_business/index.html.

Sportsman, Susan, Linda Hawley, Sharon DeBartolo Carmack, and Robin Purdy Newhouse. *Critical Practice Management Strategies for Nurse Practitioners.* Washington, DC: American Nurse's Association, 2002.

Stewart, Michael. *RN = Real News: Media Relations and You.* American Nurse's Association Continuing Education, http://nursingworld.org/mods/mod230/cernfull.htm.

Zaumeyer, Carolyn. *How to Start an Independent Practice: A Resource and Reference Manual for Nurse Practitioners.* Philadelphia: F A Davis Co., 2003.

Professional Organizations

American Academy of Physician's Assistants (http://www.aapa.org)

American Association of Nurse Anesthetists (http://www.aana.com)

American Board of Quality Assurance (http://www.abqaurp.org)

American College of Nurse Midwives (http://www.midwife.org)

American College of Nurse Practitioners (http://www.acnpweb.org)

American Nurse's Association (http://www.nursingworld.org)

Center for Medicare and Medicaid Services (http://www.cms.gov)

Joint Commission on Accreditation of Healthcare Organizations (http://www.jcaho.org)

Medical Group Management Association (http://www.mgma.com)

National Association of Pediatric Nurse Associates and Practitioners (http://www.napnap.org)

National Practitioner Data Bank (http://www.npdb-hipdb.com)

Society of Emergency Medicine Physician's Assistants (http://www.sempa.org)

GLOSSARY

Access to care The accessibility of healthcare services. Access to care may be affected by geographic constraints, a lack or shortage of healthcare providers, or insurance coverage issues.

Advanced practice nurse Registered nurse who has assumed an expanded role through education and/or experience.

Affidavit of Merit An expert's attestation that a medical malpractice case is prosecutable or defensible.

Allied healthcare provider Generic term applied to a nonphysician healthcare provider.

Bad debt write off An accounts receivable that is written off as uncollectible.

Benchmarking The continuous process of measuring services and practices against other practices. Includes the process of identifying, understanding, and adapting outstanding practices of others to improve one's own practice or performance.

Benchmarks Statistical measures used for benchmarking.

Billed revenue Revenue generated by billing clinical services.

Breach of duty Failure to adhere to the standard of care either by commission (doing something that should not have been done) or omission (failing to do something that should have been done).

Bylaws Rules of procedure for an organization.

Causation In medical malpractice it is necessary to prove that an act of omission or commission is the *cause* of an adverse outcome or injury.

Center for Medicare and Medicaid Services (CMS) Federal government agency that oversees the administration of Medicare and Medicaid health plans.

Certification Documentation of advanced education or experience obtained by a nonphysician provider. Often requires the successful completion of a national certifying examination.

Clinical nurse specialist Nurse who masters the application of nursing and related sciences to practice. Focus is usually on improved quality of care and outcomes.

Clinician Healthcare provider (for purposes of this book, clinician refers to providers who are not physicians).

Collaboration Coordination of care between a physician and a nonphysician provider.

Collaborative agreements Document that describes the legal basis for and the scope of practice of the nonphysician provider as agreed upon between the nonphysician provider and the consulting physician.

Constituent Person who lives within the voting district of a lawmaker.

Consult The act of seeking the advice or opinion of another healthcare provider.

Consultation The process of rendering an opinion at the request of another healthcare provider.

Contract Document that describes mutual agreements between individual(s).

Contractual allowances Agreed upon discounts for the provision of services to a defined group as described in the contract.

Core competencies Skills considered necessary to be mastered at the completion of an education program.

Cost measures Benchmarks that evaluate financial measures of a practice.

Counseling Service provided for the purpose of education or instruction that does not include a physical examination.

Credentialing The process of obtaining privileges from an organization or insurance company.

Current Procedural Terminology (CPT) Numeric billing codes that define a service, device, or procedure.

Curriculum Vitae Biographical outline of one's academic and professional experience, including professional memberships, honors, awards, research, and publications.

Departicipate Discontinue to accept payment from or participate with an insurance company.

Disruptive Innovator Innovation that challenges the status quo (i.e., nonphysician provider).

Duty Obligation to perform a service.

Employee handbook/manual Publication that describes human resources or personnel policies of an organization.

Evaluation and Management (E&M) Codes CPT codes that define a service provided according to the amount of history, physical exam, and medical decision making that occurred and is supported by documentation.

Expert witness Professional who articulates and evaluates the medical standard of care in a specific situation.

Fact sheet One-page document that defines a professional practice or group and what it does.

Fraud The practice of illegal billing.

Global charges Codes used to cover a procedure and pre- and postoperative care.

Gross revenue Billed revenue before expenses.

Health Care Financing Administration (HCFA) Previous name for The Center for Medicare and Medicaid Services.

Healthcare provider Generic term for healthcare professionals, including physicians and nonphysicians.

Health maintenance Wellness care, including screening, preventive counseling, education, and risk factor reduction.

Incident to billing Billing for services provided by a nonphysician provider in the name of a physician.

International Classification of Diseases (ICD) Billing codes that establish the medical necessity for a service.

Interrogatories Written questions that a person is required to answer with respect to a lawsuit.

J codes Billing codes for materials or devices.

Joint Commission for the Accreditation of Healthcare Organizations (JCAHO) Independent accrediting body for hospitals.

Legal basis for practice Authority to practice as described by federal and state law.

Liability insurance Insurance that covers a healthcare provider in the event that he or she is sued for medical malpractice.

License Document issued by the state that may be required for a healthcare provider to practice in that state.

Lobbyist A person who works on behalf of a group to support the group's political agenda.

Malpractice insurance *See* liability insurance.

Managed care Insurance company that contracts care and the reimbursement for services according to a defined set of regulations. The focus is on primary or preventive care using the primary care provider as a gatekeeper through which one must coordinate access to specialty services.

Marketing Advertising that is done to sell a product or service.

Medicaid State-administered federal health insurance program for disabled and low-income persons.

Medical Group Management Association (MGMA) Private organization that compiles and publishes data on productivity and salaries of its members according to area of clinical specialty. Widely used for benchmarking of practices.

Medical necessity The diagnosis, symptom, or complaint that is the reason for the provision of a service.

Medicare Federal health insurance program for the elderly and disabled.

Midlevel provider Generic term applied to nonphysician healthcare providers.

Modifiers Numeric two-digit codes that modify the definition of a CPT code.

Multidisciplinary healthcare team Healthcare team composed of providers from various clinical specialties.

National Data Bank An information clearinghouse established to collect and release certain information related to the professional competence and conduct of physicians, dentists, and other healthcare practitioners.

Net revenue Revenue realized by a practice after practice expenses have been deducted.

Noncompetition clause Clause in an employment contract that may prohibit the professional from working within a specified geographic area for a specified period of time so as to prevent competition with another entity.

Nonphysician provider Healthcare provider who is not a physician.

Nurse-anesthetist A registered nurse educated as an anesthesia specialist.

Nurse-midwife A nurse educated in the two disciplines of nursing and midwifery.

Nurse-practitioner Advanced practice nurse educated in a specialty area to provide health maintenance and diagnose and treat disease.

Outpatient visits Billable service provided by a clinician in an outpatient setting.

Paraprofessional Generic term applied to nonphysician healthcare providers.

Participate (par) Situation in which the healthcare provider or practice signs an agreement to participate with an insurance plan to provide services.

Patient encounter Billable service provided by a clinician for a patient.

Patient satisfaction Measurement of a patient's satisfaction with a service provided.

Payor Insurance company or other entity with whom a healthcare provider may contract with for payment of services.

Peer review Process of quality management in which healthcare professionals evaluate one another according to the accepted standards of care.

Period of discovery Phase of malpractice litigation in which both sides prepare their case.

Physician extender Generic term applied to nonphysician healthcare providers.

Physician's assistant Healthcare professionals licensed to practice medicine with physician supervision.

Political Action Committee (PAC) Group representing the legislative agenda of a specific group or organization.

Position statement Political action document that defines a problem, states the group's position on the problem, and explains how the group wishes to impact the problem.

Practice agreements *See* collaborative agreements.

Prescriptive authority The ability, according to state law, to prescribe and/or dispense medications.

Preventative medicine visit Visit for the purpose of health screening, risk factor reduction, education, and counseling.

Process improvement Processes that are implemented and evaluated with the goal of improving a service or process.

Productivity The amount of work generated.

Professional organization Organization representing professionals of similar education or clinical specialty.

Protocol Recipe for providing a service or performing a procedure.

Public relations Marketing process that promotes a person or profession.

Quality management Process involving peer review and process improvement with the goal of maintaining or improving quality of care.

Reciprocity The portability of one's licensing between states.

Referral Transferring some or all aspects of a patient's care to another healthcare provider.

Relative Value Unit (RVU) Value assigned to a medical service based on the cost of providing the service.

Resource-Based Relative Value Scale (RBRVS) System that assigns a numeric value to medical services based on the cost of providing the service.

Resume A brief account of one's academic and professional experience.

Risk management An analysis of possible loss: the profession or technique of determining, minimizing, and preventing accidental loss in a business, for example, by taking safety measures and buying insurance.

Scope of practice Parameters of a clinician's practice determined by laws, education, environment, and experience.

Specialty Area of clinical focus or expertise.

Standard of care How a reasonable clinician with a similar background would practice in a similar situation.

Tail insurance Liability insurance that covers incidents that occurred prior to or after discontinuing coverage by an insurance carrier.

Target population Groups of persons for whom the clinician is particularly qualified or interested in providing care. Groups may be defined by age, race, gender, socioeconomic status, demographics, or medical condition.

Testimony Verbal attestation by an expert on a given subject.

V codes Billing codes that establish the medical necessity for a visit that is not for a diagnosis, complaint, or symptom. Example: preventative medicine visit or a follow-up visit.

Vicarious liability Liability assumed by a healthcare provider based on the actions of another healthcare provider.

INDEX

D

Q

R

S

T

U

V

W

Z